I0789756

Healthy Holistic Pregnancy

Take a natural and holistic approach to your pregnancy

Jesse Lane Lee, BSc, CNP

Contents

Introduction

Congratulations, you are pregnant or trying to get pregnant!

It is such a crazy, exciting, happy, overwhelming, and sometimes scary time. It is a magical experience, but there can also be a lot of pressure (that you put on yourself!) to make sure you are doing everything "right".

I was motivated to write this book because when I became pregnant I started pouring through my textbooks, course notes, and of course, the internet. I wanted to make sure I was doing everything I could to grow a happy and healthy baby. I also wanted to keep everything as natural as possible.

As a holistic nutritionist, I use holistic remedies, herbs, and supplements to cure any issues I have. I also use superfoods to prevent health issues from coming up. I kept asking my midwife if this supplement or that superfood was safe for pregnancy and she wasn't able to give me the answers I wanted. I decided to take on the task of becoming an expert on holistic pregnancy practices.

I realised I probably wasn't the only holistically minded person who was asking their midwife or doctor similar questions. I also found lots misinformation online, which can be dangerous. I put a lot of time into this book to make sure it is well researched and easy to understand. My goal is to provide you with the information you need to make an informed choice about the holistic practices you choose to apply during your pregnancy.

I am not making any recommendations in this book, just providing you with the facts so you can decide what is going to work best for your body and your baby. Everybody is different and without working with you one-on-one I cannot assess your unique situation. Before trying anything in this book, please consult with your chosen healthcare practitioner.

I always wanted to be someone who loved being pregnant. During the first trimester and when my butt muscles were causing me pain, I never thought this would be possible. As I started to treat the pregnancy symptoms I was experiencing with the natural remedies I share in this book, I started to really enjoy pregnancy. I'm not sure I can say I loved being pregnant, but I did really enjoy the experience and will totally do it again! During the end of the third trimester, I found myself looking at the 20 week pregnant mamas in my yoga class with envy knowing that they are only half way through this incredible journey to motherhood.

About The Author

Hello! I'm Jesse Lane Lee, BSc, CNP, and I am a cheerful Holistic Nutritionist, cookbook author, and media personality. I am the founder of JesseLaneWellness.com, a web based holistic nutrition practice and holistic recipe resource.

I have struggled with Irritable Bowel Syndrome and food allergies on and off for most of my life, starting when I was a baby! I knew something had to change when the Irritable Bowel Syndrome symptoms I was experiencing kicked into high gear while I was studying engineering at university. I was getting sick so often that I was constantly anxious and worrying about where the washroom was in every building or situation I found myself in.

I started my healing journey by visiting a holistic practitioner who gave me the guidance I needed to heal my leaky gut. As I gathered momentum, I became really excited about cooking healthy food and I started playing in the kitchen. I had so much fun creating allergen free recipes that the restrictive diet I was following became a source of culinary inspiration.

Today, I feel fantastic and am able to enjoy most of the foods that used to cause an unwelcome reaction.

I love to get creative in the kitchen and share holistically delicious recipes that accommodate a wide variety of food allergies, diets, and lifestyle choices.

I am the author of;

- Healthy Homemade Soups & Sandwiches,
- Healthy Fresh Salads,
- Healthy Dairy Free Desserts
- and a co-author of The Holistic In the City 21 Day Smoothie Guide.

I appear frequently on TV as a guest expert on;

- Your Morning,
- Breakfast Television,
- The Morning Show,
- Morning Live,
- Daytime Toronto,
- and several local TV shows.

I am also a regular contributor to Clean Eating Magazine, KrisCarr.com, and MindBodyGreen.com.

I believe that eating healthy whole foods can be easy, fun and most of all, delicious!

Acknowledgements

There are a few people that I wish to personally thank for helping me make this book a reality. A huge thank you to:

My Husband, who has been so caring during the pregnancy. He supported my desire for a holistic pregnancy and natural birth in so many ways. He also spent countless hours editing and designing this book and was able to meet my super short and very unreasonable deadlines.

Margot Schelew, my mom, who generously wrote a section on yoga and pregnancy explaining the benefits of prenatal yoga and providing information about which poses to avoid and modify when pregnant. Margot is a yoga teacher with prenatal training, a hypnotherapist, and a hypnobirthing instructor. Check out Margot's website at hypnosisinthecity.ca.

Andrea Ashley, who was kind enough to contribute a section on essential oil safety while pregnant. She explains which oils to avoid and shares some DIY recipes. Andrea has an education in advanced skincare, master clinical aromatherapy, diplomas in both organic skincare science and organic skincare formulation and certifications in holistic therapies. Check out Andrea's website at andreaashley.ca.

Danielle Milgrom, who did a fantastic job editing this book and helping me develop and implement the launch. Check her out on Instagram @daniellemilgromwellness

Danny Mejia, who is the fantastic photographer behind the cover of this book. He was trouper when all of the mosquitos came out during the shoot. He also did our engagement shoot, wedding, and a beach yoga photoshoot for me! Check out his website at www.dmphoto.ca

Cassandra Busuttil, who is a fantastic editor.

My midwives Grace, Nousin and my student midwife Mariah from the Midwives Collective of Toronto, who patiently answered all of my questions and inspired me to share my knowledge.

Holistic Nutrition for Pregnancy

Nutrition is so important when you are pregnant because it can make the difference between a healthy, happy pregnancy and one where you are constantly experiencing pregnancy discomforts. Getting the nourishment you and your baby needs can be done through eating a nutrient dense diet, adding superfoods to your diet, or taking supplements.

Many superfoods and supplements can have tremendous health benefits when taken during pregnancy; however often times there is insufficient information to prove that they are safe or unsafe to consume. My goal is to explain both sides of the debate and share my experience with you.

I hope that this information will allow you to make an informed decision on what is best for you and your pregnancy. Please talk to your healthcare provider before eating any of the superfoods or taking any of the supplements mentioned in this book.

Key Pregnancy Nutrients

When you are pregnant your body needs more of everything! It is working hard to support your daily activities and to grow your beautiful baby. When you are pregnant there is high demand for calories, protein, calcium, iron, and B vitamins.

<u>Calories</u>

Does eating for two mean you actually get to eat as much as you want of everything?

Unfortunately it doesn't work that way because your baby is much smaller than a child or adult. When you are pregnant, you need to consume about 20% to 25% more calories than usual depending on the trimester and your weight before becoming pregnant.

During the first trimester, your caloric needs don't really change a whole lot because your baby is so small. During the second trimester, you will need an extra 300 calories per day or more if you had a hard first trimester with morning sickness. During the third trimester you need about 450 extra calories per day. To put this in perspective, there are about 300 calories in a bowl of oatmeal and 500 calories in a bowl of chickpea pasta with sauce. If you were underweight before becoming pregnant your caloric intake will be a bit higher, and if you were overweight your caloric intake will be lower.

It is important to make these calories count by consuming nutrient dense foods as opposed to junk food you might be craving.

<u>Protein</u>

Pregnant women need about 50% more protein during pregnancy, which translates to 70 to 85 grams of protein per day. Protein is really important because it is the building block of your baby's body. Protein supports tissue growth of the baby and the new tissues you are growing to support birth.

The most nutrient dense sources of protein are:
- Cod
- Shrimp
- Turkey
- Chicken
- Beef
- Lamb
- Sardines
- Tofu
- Soybeans or edamame
- Yogurt
- Lentils
- High quality plant based protein powders

All animal sources of protein and soy based products on this list should be organic to reduce the amount of hormones, pesticides, and antibiotics you consume.

<u>Calcium</u>

Calcium is a bone builder, which will help your baby's bones and teeth form, aid in your baby's muscle and heart function, blood clotting, and nerve transmission. Pregnant women need about 1,300mg of calcium per day.

If you don't consume enough calcium, your body will start

pulling it from your bones to nourish your baby. This can cause decreased bone strength and may trigger toxins to be pulled from your bones and passed on to your baby.

The most nutrient dense sources of calcium are:
- Spinach
- Collard greens
- Basil
- Yogurt
- Milk
- Cheese
- Sesame seeds
- Swiss chard
- Tofu

Iron

When you are pregnant your blood volume increases by 50%, so the demand for iron goes up by 50%. Iron is an extremely important nutrient during pregnancy because it is needed to build you and your baby's blood cells. Iron also helps keep your energy levels high and helps keep your immune system strong. Pregnant women need 27mg of iron per day.

The most nutrient dense sources of iron are:
- Meat and poultry
- Spinach
- Swiss chard
- Tofu
- Shiitake mushrooms
- Shrimp
- Soybeans
- Olives
- Lentils

- Pumpkin seeds
- Sesame seeds
- Quinoa
- Kidney beans
- Blackstrap molasses

Iron is more easily absorbed when eaten with a food rich in vitamin C, like bell peppers, parsley, broccoli, strawberries, cauliflower, citrus, and papaya.

<u>Folic acid aka folate or vitamin B9</u>

Folic acid is the most important B vitamin during pregnancy and before conception because it helps prevent neural tube defects. It also helps with the formation of red blood cells, aids in the growth and reproduction of cells, and supports your baby's nervous system development. Pregnant women need 400 to 600mcg per day.

The most nutrient dense sources of folic acid are:
- Spinach
- Asparagus
- Celery
- Pinto beans
- Black beans
- Chickpeas
- Kidney beans
- Navy beans
- Liver

Pregnancy Power Foods

Your healthcare provider will likely have told you which regular foods you should avoid while pregnant. This is something you can easily look up online if you haven't already.

When you are pregnant it is important to eat a healthy diet so you can support yourself and your growing baby. During the first trimester this might be tough if you have food aversions, but try to eat as many of these pregnancy power foods as you can.

Dark leafy green veggies

Dark leafy green veggies like spinach, kale, Swiss chard and other greens are fantastic for pregnancy. They are packed with essential pregnancy nutrients like vitamin A, C, and K. They also contain folate which is an important nutrient that reduces the risk of neural tube defects. Consuming green, leafy vegetables has also been linked to a reduced risk of low birth weight. (7, 8)

During the first trimester you might not be able to eat salads, so I recommend adding greens to your smoothies, or pureeing them and adding them to pasta sauce or other meals. Once you are able to eat regularly again, greens can be added to eggs, soup, sandwiches, stir fry, enjoyed as a side dish, and in salad. Try my Blueberry Ginger Smoothie Recipe on page 90 or Green Eggs on page 95.

Nuts and seeds

Nuts and seeds are an excellent source of omega-3s, which

is great for you and your baby's brain health. They are also high in fibre and protein which are both important for pregnancy. Fibre will make sure things keep moving since constipation is common. Protein is super important for your baby's development. It is safe to eat peanuts and nuts during pregnancy as long as you are not allergic.

I like to enjoy nuts and seeds as a protein packed energy boosting snack. You can also sprinkle them over yoghurt, oatmeal, cereal, salads, and stir-fry's and enjoy them in trail mix. Try my Superfood Trail Mix Recipe on page 100.

Legumes

I love beans for pregnancy, because similar to nuts and seeds, they are high in fibre and protein. When you are pregnant your digestive system slows down and many women experience constipation and hemorrhoids. Eating high fibre foods is a great way to keep things moving well. Beans are also high in important pregnancy nutrients like iron, folate, calcium, and zinc.

There are so many different types of legumes and so many ways to enjoy them! Chickpeas are awesome roasted or made into hummus. Lentils are fantastic in soups or mixed into rice and I love sprinkling black beans and navy beans over my salads. Try my hummus recipe on page 98, Crispy Chickpea recipe on page 99, and Bean Salad recipe on page 103.

Eggs

Eggs are a protein powerhouse and contain lots of vitamins and minerals. Protein is so important during pregnancy because your baby's cells are growing like crazy and protein is the main building block for those cells. Eggs are also high in choline, which promotes baby's overall growth and brain health.

When eating eggs, some people recommend making sure they are cooked through, even the yolk. Eggs make a fantastic breakfast, you can enjoy them scrambled or in an omelet. Hardboiled eggs make a great snack and they can be added to a salad. Try my Green Eggs on page 95 and my Gluten-free Quiche recipe on page 96.

Blackstrap Molasses

Blackstrap molasses has very little sugar content giving it a robust and bittersweet flavor which is very different from Fancy Molasses. It is rich in iron, which transports oxygen from the lungs to all cells in the body and it plays a key role in energy production and metabolism. With all of the extra blood circulating your body, iron is super important. Blackstrap molasses also contains a significant amount of calcium.

The tastiest way to enjoy molasses is in baking with ginger! My mom likes to eat it over toast with nut butter. You can also drizzle it over oatmeal or add it to savoury sauces. Try my Carrot Molasses Muffin recipe on page 93.

Nutritional Yeast

Nutritional Yeast is rich in folate, vitamin B12, and iron, all of which are important nutrients for you and your baby. Folate helps prevent major birth defects like spina bifida and 1 Tbsp of nutritional yeast meets your daily needs. Vitamin B12 is necessary for healthy development of your baby and iron is needed to keep your energy levels high.

I am totally addicted to nutritional yeast! It has a zesty flavour which is cheese like. You can sprinkle it anywhere you would use parmesan cheese or use it in sauces. I use it in my pesto recipe on page 109.

Yogurt

Good quality organic yogurt is an excellent food to enjoy while pregnant because it is packed with probiotics. Probiotics are really important to keep your digestive system healthy, boost your immune system which tends to be weak during pregnancy, and reduce the chance of vaginal and urinary tract infections. Organic Greek yogurt is also a fantastic source of protein.

If you follow a dairy free diet, you can find delicious coconut and almond yogurts at big grocery stores and health food stores.

I generally follow a dairy free diet, but I found myself craving plain organic Greek yogurt during my pregnancy, so I enjoyed it a few times a week. I love having yogurt bowls for breakfast topped with fresh berries, chia seeds, and granola. If you are eating coconut or almond yogurt, you might want to stir in some plant based protein powder or collagen powder to increase the protein content.

Bone Broth

Bone broth is a pregnancy superfood because it is packed with minerals that are essential to you and your baby's health. It is high in gelatin and collagen, and contains protein and healthy fats. These nutrients will help grow your baby's bones, cartilage, connective tissues, and joints.

If you are experiencing nausea and having a hard time eating, bone broth is a great way to get some nutrients into your body and to keep you hydrated. It is also a great drink to sip on during labour.

I like making my own bone broth, you can find my recipe on page 107. If the smell of bone broth cooking bothers you there are lots of pre-made versions that you can find at health food stores or online. Just make sure you are getting bone broth and not beef stock, there is a huge difference in the mineral content. I like to drink it warmed up or use it in soups and stews.

<u>Salmon</u>

Being from the east coast I love fish and salmon is one of my favourites. Salmon is really high in omega-3 fatty acids which are essential during pregnancy. Omega-3s help build baby's brain and eyes. If you find you are experiencing baby brain, omega-3s will also help you as well!

When pregnant, you may want to limit your intake of fish because it can be high in mercury. While I was pregnant (after the first trimester when I could stand the smell of fish again) I tried to consume salmon once a week but I also took an Omega-3 supplement with EPA and DHA.

Try my Kale Oregano Pesto Salmon recipe on page 109.

Organic Meat

Protein and iron are super important during pregnancy and
meat is one of the best sources of both nutrients. Lots of
protein is needed because it is the building block of your
growing baby's cells. Iron is important because it is found
in red blood cells as a part of the hemoglobin that delivers
oxygen to all of the cells in the body. Low level of iron
during pregnancy can lead to premature delivery and low
birth weight which is something we all want to avoid.

During the first trimester you might have an aversion to meat
like I did. In this case it is important to get your protein and
iron from the plant-based foods mentioned on page 6.

During the second and third trimester it should be easier
to eat meat several times a week, if not every day. When
cooking meat, it is important to cook it all the way through
to make sure that any bacteria in the meat are killed. I highly
recommend buying organic meat to avoid hormones, antibiotics, and the other downfalls of factory farmed meat.

Whole Grains

Whole grains are great to enjoy during pregnancy because
they are packed with fibre and vitamins. Fibre is important
during pregnancy because your digestive system can get
sluggish which leads to constipation. Fibre is a great way to
keep everything moving smoothly. Whole grains are generally
rich in B-vitamins, which are essential during pregnancy
because they help with baby's brain and nervous system
development and they will keep your energy levels high.

My favourite whole grains are quinoa, oats, and brown rice.

Quinoa is a super versatile grain that is also high in protein. I like to eat it for breakfast, in my salads, and as a side with my dinner. Oats make an excellent fibre packed breakfast and rice is fantastic with dinner. Try my recipe for Breakfast Quinoa on page 91 and Mediterranean Quinoa Salad on page 105.

Superfoods

I found there was a big gap in the information available about which superfoods to avoid when pregnant. I would ask my midwife and sometimes she hadn't heard of the superfood before.

I decided to do some of my own research and share it with you. This is no way a complete list. If something is missing from this list, it doesn't mean that it is safe to consume when pregnant, it just means I didn't think of adding it!

It is really important to talk to your healthcare provider before eating any superfoods when pregnant.

<u>Bee Products</u>

Honey is one of my favourite natural sweeteners because it is rich in enzymes, minerals, and antioxidants. It has incredible healing properties and is antibacterial, antimicrobial, and antiviral. I also love using propolis spray when I have a sore throat or feel a cold coming on.

It is not safe for babies to consume honey because it can cause botulism, but it is a different story for expecting mamas. Your digestive tract is much more acidic than your baby's and it contains a healthy bacterium that prevents the honey spores from developing into botulism-causing bacteria. Since you are the one eating the honey, your digestive tract will kill any bad bacteria before the honey reaches your bloodstream and your baby.

There really isn't any research on the safety of other bee products like propolis, bee pollen, or royal jelly. In general, if you have a bee allergy or seasonal allergies, it is best to avoid bee products as they can cause an allergic reaction. I highly recommend talking to your healthcare provider before consuming raw honey, propolis, bee pollen, or royal jelly.

I decided to consume raw honey and propolis while pregnant because they were both part of my regular diet beforehand and I have a close relationship with my beekeeper.

<u>Dandelion Root</u>

Dandelion roots can help improve digestion, relieve constipation, and soothe an upset stomach. Dandelions are also a liver tonic that detoxify the liver and ease congestion in the liver which can cause morning sickness. They also help purify the bladder and kidneys and reduce the risk of urinary tract infections, which are important to avoid when pregnant as they can lead to preterm labour.

Although dandelion is generally considered safe, no formal safety studies have been done on women who are pregnant or nursing. Talk to your healthcare provider before consuming dandelion root as a supplement or in mass amounts.

I am a big fan of dandelion root tea and the powdered dandelion root coffee substitute. I drank it from time to time while pregnant when I was craving that coffee flavour.

<u>Elderberry</u>

Elderberry juice is a powerful immune booster that can reduce cold and flu symptoms and protect the body from sinus infections.

Like many natural superfoods, elderberry juice and syrup have not undergone enough research to consider them safe to consume when pregnant.

<u>Green tea</u>

Green tea is often considered a superfood due to its high antioxidant content. There is increased oxidative stress during pregnancy so antioxidants provide much needed cellular protection for you and your baby.

The problem with green tea is that it contains caffeine. Caffeine consumption during pregnancy could increase the risk of miscarriage or low birth weight which can lead to other health issues down the road. Most doctors agree that 200mg of caffeine per day is safe. An 8oz cup of green tea contains 24mg to 45mg so one or two cups a day could be considered safe.

I found caffeine made me nauseous during pregnancy so I typically avoided it. When I wanted to drink a caffeinated tea I would steep it for 30 seconds, pour out the tea, then steep for the recommended time. Some claim that this removes 80% of the caffeine, but I couldn't find any reputable studies to back this up. I did find it worked for me in terms of preventing nausea, but it could be the placebo effect.

<u>Goji Berries</u>

Goji berries are amazing because they are so nutrient rich. They contain amino acids, antioxidants, vitamins, minerals, and important trace minerals. They strengthen the immune system and boost energy levels.

Again, there is not a lot of research on the safety of goji berries while pregnant. One thing to consider is that goji berries are loosely linked to miscarriages because they can cause uterine contractions. I also found that if you are taking anticoagulants to prevent blood clots, you want to check with your healthcare provider first.

Personally, I had goji berries from time to time while I was pregnant but I never had more than a few at a time. If you are a goji berry lover, please talk to your healthcare provider before making a decision.

<u>Kombucha</u>

If you followed me on social media or read my blog before I became pregnant, you will know that I'm totally obsessed with kombucha and used to make my own weekly. Kombucha is awesome for your digestion because it is rich in probiotics and enzymes that nourish the digestive tract. It also boosts metabolism, detoxifies the liver, and contains energy boosting B vitamins.

There are three issues with consuming kombucha when pregnant; alcohol content, caffeine, and risk of bad bacteria. Kombucha is a fermented drink, so naturally it has an alcohol content of 1%-3%, non-alcoholic beer is around 0.5%. Kombucha is also made with caffeinated tea and caffeine intake should be regulated while pregnant. Finally, if you are new to making kombucha at home, there is a risk of your culture developing bad bacteria or mould that can harm your baby.

Personally, I stopped making my own kombucha while pregnant because I knew I would always be stressing over the smell and health of my culture. I didn't consume store bought kombucha too often because after you make your own for 0.25$/500ml it is really hard to pay $5 or more at the grocery store!

Medicinal Mushrooms

Medicinal mushrooms like Reishi, Chaga, and Cylocepts are getting really popular due to their incredible healing ability. They are excellent cancer fighters and they are adaptogenic, which means that they will go to work wherever the body needs extra help.

The problem is there isn't a lot of research around the safety of consuming medical mushrooms when pregnant. On top of that, the way the mushrooms are harvested is a cause for concern because they are usually picked from the wild and are not overly regulated.

If you do wish to consume medicinal mushrooms during your pregnancy, I recommend talking to your healthcare provider or a traditional Chinese medicine doctor before proceeding. Personally I choose not to consume medicinal mushrooms while pregnant.

MTC Oil

MTC Oil is processed in the liver and quickly absorbed to provide fast and sustained energy which is great when you are feeling sluggish.

As with many superfoods, there isn't sufficient research to support the safety of MCT oil when pregnant. Although MCT oil has a ton of health benefits, there is evidence that medium chain triglycerides can deplete essential fatty acids in your baby.

To be on the safe side you may want to avoid MCT oil when pregnant. If you are looking for a good substitute, use regular coconut oil which still has all of the immune boosting antibacterial properties and healthy fats.

<u>Moringa</u>

Moringa leaves are high in calcium which is important for you and your baby's bones, choline which prevents spinal cord and brain defects, and folic acid which controls spinal cord defects. This is a bit of a controversial superfood because Moringa leaves have a ton of health benefits but the roots, stems, seeds, and flowers can be dangerous.

Moringa roots and stems have actually been used as a contraceptive and used to cause miscarriages. They have been found to prevent the fertilized egg from attaching to the lining of the uterine wall. The seeds, roots, and stems can also contain immunosuppressive and cytotoxic effects that you definitely want to avoid. (9, 10, 11, 12)

Some sources claim that the leaves can have the same properties as the roots and stems. For this reason, I decided not to take moringa while pregnant or while I was trying to conceive.

<u>Protein Powder</u>

Protein is the building block for you and your baby's cells. You need more protein when you are pregnant to support your own body and your growing baby. Protein intake is especially important in the third trimester when your baby is growing really quickly. A great way to add more protein into your diet is with protein powder.

Many of my favourite protein powder brands have warnings against use when pregnant or breastfeeding because they contain some of the controversial superfoods and supplements mentioned in this book. They may also contain added vitamins that could bring you above the recommended daily amount.

Your best bet is to carefully read the labels. Look for a clean plant-based protein powder with no added sugar that only contains one protein source and no additional superfoods, supplements, or enzymes.

<u>Sprouts</u>

Sprouting beans is a great way to make them more digestible and increase their nutrient content. Beans contain a protective layer of phytic acid and enzyme inhibitors that make them really difficult for us to digest. Soaking your beans neutralizes both of these guys. Beans also contain complex sugars that many people struggle to digest, leaving them to ferment and feed bad bacteria in the digestive tract. Sprouting beans breaks down these complex sugars so our bodies don't have to.

The big problem with sprouting beans at home or buying sprouts is contamination. Bacteria like salmonella, listeria, and E.coli can get into seeds or beans through cracks in the shell and can continue to grow as they sprout. These food borne illnesses can be found in both store bought and homemade sprouts and could lead to miscarriages, stillbirth, or premature birth.

Cooking sprouts will kill any bacteria that you are worried about. You can still get the digestive benefits of sprouting beans if you cook them after they are sprouted. You will lose some of the enzymes but they will still have lots of protein and fibre. The only sprouts that don't fall into this category are Brussel sprouts which you can enjoy raw.

Safe Superfoods
- Acai berry – Unless you have a food allergy, Acai berry is safe during pregnancy. It is a nutrient-dense fruit that contains amino acids that promote your baby's growth. It is also packed with vitamins, minerals, and antioxidants that will keep you and baby healthy.
- Flax, hemp, and chia seeds – All of these seeds are rich in bowel regulating fibre, baby building protein, and brain supporting omega-3 fatty acids.
- Raw cacao – Raw cacao powder and nibs are packed with free radical fighting antioxidants, blood boosting iron, and relaxing magnesium. Cacao does contain a little bit of caffeine so don't go too crazy!
- Sea vegetables – Kelp, nori, Dulse, and all other forms of sea vegetables are packed with iodine which is important for your thyroid health and metabolism. It can also boost your baby's IQ.

Supplements

This in no way a complete list of supplements; I tried to cover the most popular supplements my clients were taking. If something is missing from this list, it doesn't mean that it is safe to consume when pregnant, it just means I didn't think of adding it! I would be so grateful if you could email info@jesselanewellness.com to let me know what is missing so I can add it to future editions or share it in a blog post.

It is really important to always read the labels of your supplements and talk to your healthcare provider before taking ANY supplement when pregnant.

While I was pregnant, I took probiotics, prenatal vitamins, fish oil, and a calcium + magnesium + D3 supplement daily. I also had a pregnancy specific digestive enzyme for meals that I knew my body would struggle to digest. This combo worked really well for me because I have underlying digestive issues, but you might need to take a totally different handful of supplements depending on what health issues you were experiencing before getting pregnant. A qualified holistic nutritionist like me or naturopathic doctor can help you determine which supplements are best for you and your baby's needs. That being said, you can't go wrong with a good quality prenatal vitamin.

Activated Charcoal

Activated charcoal is an excellent detoxifier and is very effective at treating food poisoning. During pregnancy, many women experience morning sickness that can be due to elevated toxins the body is trying to eliminate. Activated charcoal consumption during pregnancy could reduce morning sickness, keep the body energized, and boost your mood.

The body does not digest charcoal; therefore it does not collect in your bloodstream. The Mayo Clinic states that activated charcoal has not been reported to cause birth defects or other problems in humans during pregnancy; however it is always a good idea to check with your healthcare provider before taking it.

Activated charcoal wasn't a part of my diet before pregnancy and my morning sickness was mild, so I didn't add it to my diet once I became pregnant.

<u>Adaptogens</u>

I often use adaptogenic herbs like ashwagandha, astragalus, ginseng, holy basil, licorice root, maca, and rhodiola to help regulate my client's stress levels. They work by supporting the adrenal glands which are in charge of managing stress hormones.

When you are pregnant, your hormone levels are all over the place as they adjust to your growing baby. It is advisable not to take anything that may alter your hormone levels which naturally change during pregnancy.

In addition to that:
- Ashwaganda causes spasmolytic activity in the uterus which can cause abortion when consumed in large quantities.
- Certain species of astragalus are great for strengthening expecting momma's immune systems,

but others can lead to miscarriages or birth defects.
- Ginseng can help with energy levels and boost the immune system, tulsi can help manage stress, and rhodiola is used to better cope with stress; however there isn't sufficient information to determine if they are safe or unsafe during pregnancy.
- Licorice root is great for regulating stress levels however it has been linked to premature labor when taken in large doses. Licorice root is often found in teas to add sweetness so make sure you read your labels.
- Maca is used to balance hormones levels, some consider it safe during pregnancy and others do not. It is a staple in the diets of pregnant and nursing Peruvian women.

I decided to avoid all adaptogens while I was pregnant.

Chlorella

Chlorella is a blue-green algae that is bursting with nutrients that are perfect for pregnancy. It contains folate, vitamin B12, and iron and can reduce the effect of swelling or edema during pregnancy. In addition to that, there was a study done in Japan (12) that found taking chlorella during pregnancy can reduce dioxin levels in breast milk. This is important because dioxin is an environmental contaminant that we do not want to pass along to our babies.

Like most supplements, sources are divided on the safety of chlorella during pregnancy because the Japanese study seems to be the only one available.

Chlorella wasn't a part of my diet before pregnancy, so I

didn't add it to my diet once I became pregnant.

<u>Collagen</u>

Collagen helps build and repair our bones, joints, and is important for skin health. It can help reduce stretch marks and provide our body and growing baby with essential protein.

Collagen supplements are usually derived from animals or fish, so it is important to look for a brand that offers grass-fed, pasture-raised, sustainably raised animals or wild-caught fish. You also want to make sure you are getting 100% collagen without any fillers or additives.

During the first trimester I had trouble eating animal products, so I really liked mixing collagen powder into the almond milk I pour over my granola, into coconut yoghurt, and apple sauce.

<u>CoQ10</u>

Coenzyme Q10 is an antioxidant found naturally in the body. It supports the cardiovascular system and helps with energy production at a cellular level. There was a study done (13) that found that supplementation with CoQ10 during pregnancy reduces the risk of developing pre-eclampsia (high blood pressure) in women at risk for the condition.

Despite this study, many still believe that there is a lack of scientific evidence on the use of CoQ10 during pregnancy or breastfeeding. Please talk to a qualified professional before adding it to your supplement regime.

Curcumin

The bright yellow/orange pigment of turmeric called curcumin has been shown to be comparable to potent drugs such as hydrocortisone and over-the-counter anti-inflammatory drugs. It is effective in the treatment of inflammatory bowel disease, rheumatoid arthritis, and cystic fibrosis due to its antioxidant concentrations and anti-inflammatory properties.

There are some concerns of high levels of curcumin stimulating the uterus and causing premature birth and miscarriages.

If you are looking to benefit from the anti-inflammatory properties of curcumin, stick to turmeric in its whole form instead of taking a supplement. You can enjoy it in curries and soups. I liked to drink turmeric ginger tea during pregnancy whenever I felt a cold coming on.

Digestive Enzymes

If you are someone who struggled with your digestion before becoming pregnant, chances are it will not get any better once you are actually pregnant because your digestive system will slow down even more. If you didn't have digestive issues before pregnancy and are experiencing them now, digestive enzymes may not be the answer, but we will cover that later in this book.

It has been stated that some enzymes like pancreatin should not be taken during pregnancy.

Make sure you read the bottle of your enzymes to make

sure they do not contain a warning for pregnant women. I ended up purchasing a digestive enzyme that is specifically formulated for pregnancy.

<u>Echinacea</u>

When you are pregnant your body can be more susceptible to colds. Echinacea is an herbal supplement used to prevent colds and to reduce their length.

A Motherisk study (14) showed that use of echinacea during the first trimester of pregnancy was not associated with increased risk of major malformations. This was a small study and is not enough to deem Echinacea safe for pregnant women.

I took a high quality Echinacea tincture a few times during my pregnancy when I felt like I was coming down with a cold.

<u>Herbs</u>

Herbs can have amazing healing powers and can be used in teas, tonics, tinctures, and more.

There are several herbs that can stimulate the uterus causing contractions that can trigger a miscarriage. The most common herbs to avoid when pregnant are:
- Aloe Vera (externally is OK)
- Angelica
- Autumn crocus
- Arum
- Barberry
- Birthwort
- Black Cohosh

- Blessed Thistle
- Buckthorn
- Don Quai
- Ephedra
- Ginseng
- Goldenseal
- Gotu Cola
- Juniper
- Male Fern
- Mandrake
- Passion Flower
- Pennyroyal
- Poke Root
- Rue
- Saffron
- Sage
- Southernwood
- Tansy
- Thuja
- Wormwood

I generally avoided herbs while pregnant unless they were found in teas. Always check with a qualified herbalist before taking any herbs when pregnant, even if they are not on this list.

<u>Milk Thistle</u>

During pregnancy your hormones are raging and sometimes the liver can struggle to eliminate excess hormones and toxins which can contribute to morning sickness. Milk thistle supports the liver detox process and can alleviate morning sickness.

Milk thistle has been used historically to improve the flow of breast milk and a limited study on pregnant women reported a lack of side effects. However, there is lack of evidence to support the safe use of milk thistle while pregnant so check with you healthcare provider before taking it.

Oil of oregano

Oil of oregano is a very powerful antimicrobial, antiviral, and antibacterial making it an excellent way to fight colds and flus. It also contains antifungal properties that help fight candida and yeast infections.

Oil of oregano should not be used during pregnancy because it promotes menstrual flow, which can increase the risk of miscarriage.

Although oil of oregano is dangerous, it is ok to use small amounts of fresh or dried herbs in your cooking.

Spirulina

Iron deficiency is really common during pregnancy due to an increased blood volume. Low iron can make you feel super sluggish and tired. Spirulina is a blue-green algae that is an excellent source of easily digestible iron that is less likely to cause constipation. It is also a complete protein source which is important for your growing baby.

With spirulina powder, there is a risk of heavy metal contamination so you want to make sure you buy a clean brand that you trust. Unfortunately, there is not enough scientific information about consuming spirulina during pregnancy to determine whether using it while pregnant or breast-feeding is safe.

Vitamin A, D, E and K

Vitamin A is essential for the growth of your baby and plays an important role in baby's hearing, vision, and heart health. Vitamin D needs increase during pregnancy to accommodate baby's bone development. The most absorbable form is vitamin D3. Vitamin E helps get oxygen to the cells and protects RNA and DNA from damage which could result in congenital birth defects. Vitamin K is made by good gut bacteria and helps with blood clotting.

If you are taking a prenatal vitamin and eating a healthy diet, you are probably getting enough of these four vitamins and should not be supplementing separately. Since these vitamins are fat soluble, they are stored in your body for long periods of time and toxicity can happen when they are taken in excess. Too much vitamin A can cause birth defects in the developing fetus so you want to make sure you aren't getting more than the required amount of 770 micrograms daily or 2,300 IU; anything over 3,000 micrograms is dangerous.

I was really happy with the quality of the prenatal that I was taking 3 times a day and did not feel the need to take extra vitamins.

Vitamin C

As you probably know, vitamin C does a great job boosting the immune system and keeping colds away. This is beneficial when you are pregnant because often your immune system is a little weaker than usual. Vitamin C is also needed to make collagen which will help your baby grow, keep the protective membrane around your baby strong, and help prevent stretch marks. Finally, vitamin C helps with the absorption of much needed iron.

When taken in excess, vitamin C when can cause pre-term labour, rebound scurvy, and dry up cervical mucous. It is not recommended to take vitamin C supplements when pregnant. If you are taking a prenatal vitamin and eating a healthy diet you should be getting enough vitamin C to support your immune system and collagen production.

First Trimester

The first trimester is from week 1 to week 12. The thing that surprised me was that week 1 starts on the first day of your last period so you aren't actually pregnant week 1 and 2!

The first trimester of pregnancy was exciting, scary, and overwhelming at the same time! It is such a weird time, because you are going through major changes but usually your partner is the only person who knows. You spend a lot of time trying to act normal and hide your excitement and pregnancy symptoms.

I had elaborate plans on how I was going to announce to my husband that I'm pregnant, but in the end I was too excited to keep it in! I basically told him I had a feeling I was pregnant because I was a couple days late so I took a pregnancy test. After the 2 minutes were up I ran out of the bathroom yelling "I told you so" while waving the pregnancy test in his face. It wasn't the heartwarming surprise I had planned but it was pretty memorable and funny.

The first thing we did after we finished celebrating was apply to get a midwife. In Toronto, midwives are in high demand and I didn't want to risk not getting one. After that, we called our parents to share the good news with them.

We decided not to wait to tell our close friends because we figured if something happened we would want their support.

We had so much fun slowly sharing the news with friends in silly ways whenever we saw them. Friends would offer me a drink and I would casually say "No thank you, I won't be drinking for the next 9 months". It was funny because sometimes it would take a while for it to click. My friends know I like to do cleanses and abstain from alcohol from time to time so turning down a drink wasn't uncommon. My husband also liked to joke that he has a DD for the next 9 months. We also deliberately left baby books and shoes around the house so when friends were over they would see them, get a funny expression on their face, and finally ask "umm do you guys have news?".

The Bump

During the first trimester I didn't really have a bump so I was able to wear my regular clothes most of the time. By week 12 I only gained 4lbs so it wasn't noticeable. Near the end of the trimester, my tighter skinny jeans started getting a little tight so sometimes I would unbutton them when I sat down or use a hair elastic to keep them up instead of buttoning them.

Favourite things about the 1st trimester

My husband was so excited about the pregnancy and super sweet. When I mentioned I was craving something, he would go out and pick it up right away. He was also amazing to put up with all of my food aversions and made me meals I could stomach because even preparing food made me nauseous.

I also really enjoyed telling our friends and family. Everyone was so excited and sometimes people became emotional over the news which made me emotional all over again.

<u>Exercise</u>

I didn't change my exercise regime too much during the first trimester. I continued to walk my dog for an hour a day and go to yoga 3 times a week. I stayed away from the hot yoga classes and I made sure I wasn't doing any deep twisting or inversions. I learned that it is really important to let your yoga teacher know you are pregnant in the early stages because there are some poses that will cause spotting and are potentially dangerous to your baby. This was really weird because my yoga family at the studio knew I was pregnant before a bunch of my friends and family members.

<u>Cravings</u>

During the first trimester I experienced so many food aversions. Anything that didn't make me want to barf could be classified as a craving! Around week 6 the food aversions set in and I found I could no longer eat certain foods and forcing myself to eat them anyways was not an option.

The foods I craved where:
- Pizza
- Pasta
- Veggie and hummus
- Fries
- Smoothies
- Dim sum
- Apples and nut butter
- Fruit; like berries, watermelon and pineapple
- Apple Sauce

Mood

I was lucky to be in a really good mood for most of the first trimester. I think I was just so happy to be pregnant! I wasn't overly emotional and didn't have mood swings.

I tried really hard not to constantly worry about my baby's health. We opted out of the 7 week ultrasound so we didn't get confirmation that there was actually a healthy baby in there until we heard the heartbeat around the 11 week mark. Every little bit of spotting or cramping sensation totally freaked me out but I got better at not worrying so much.

Sleep

Sleeping in the first trimester was the same as always. I could sleep in any position I wanted to and got a solid 7-8 hours every night. I did find I would get super tired around 3pm so I started napping which allowed me to be more alert at night, especially if we had something fun planned with friends.

Healthcare

In Ontario we are really lucky because midwife care is covered by the government. The midwife model of care really resonated with me and I had a bunch of friends who had very positive experiences with midwives, so I knew I wanted to work with a midwife. I also wanted a natural birth at the Birthing Centre rather than at a hospital, so working with a midwife was the way to go. During the first trimester we visited our midwife on a monthly basis and got to know her and our secondary midwife really well.

<u>What I was happy to leave behind</u>

Food aversions and nausea that I experienced during the
first trimester are something I will not miss. I started feeling
car sick sometime between 2 pm and 4 pm every afternoon
and it would usually last until 9 pm. I think it was sheer will
that I didn't actually throw up. Some evenings I would spend
the whole night on the couch groaning and hoping that TV
would distract me so I wouldn't barf. It was such a relief
when this passed so I could actually like food again and to get
back into the kitchen after avoiding it for 2 months.

I was also happy to leave behind super tender boobs. My
boobs hurt SO MUCH during the first trimester. So much
that I had to wear a bra to bed because it hurt when I moved
around from one side to another. This was a weird shift for
me because I usually don't wear a bra when I'm home, which
is most of the time since I work from home! It also made
some yoga poses and hugs really uncomfortable.

Key Supplements

Vitamin D

Vitamin D is important because it will make sure you have a strong immune system and it will contribute to your baby's vitamin D stores and bone development. You can get a lot of vitamin D from safe sun exposure in the summer. If it is winter time you may want to supplement with vitamin D3 drops.

Iron

Iron is an important nutrient during pregnancy because it is needed to build you and your baby's blood cells. Iron also helps keep your energy levels high and keep your immune system strong. If you follow a vegan or vegetarian diet, you may want to get your iron level tested by your healthcare provider to see if you would benefit from iron supplementation. It is usually standard to test iron levels in the third trimester.

Folic Acid

Folic acid is the most important B vitamin during pregnancy and before conception because it helps prevent neural tube defects. It also helps with the formation of red blood cells, aids in the growth and reproduction of cells, and supports your baby's nervous system development. Most prenatal vitamins have adequate amounts of folic acid, however if you weren't getting enough folic acid before becoming pregnant you may want to add an extra vitamin B9 to your daily regime.

Common discomforts and how to treat them naturally

Acne and other skin issues

With your hormones constantly changing, skin problems like acne, red marks, and dark blotches on your face are very common. They usually disappear with the birth of your baby but who wants to wait 9 months for zits to go away!

Acne and skin issue suggestions:
- Keep your skin clean.
- Switch to clean cosmetic products and makeup that do not contain chemicals and toxins that can irritate the skin. My favourite moisturiser is coconut oil.
- Get adequate folic acid, this can also help with skin problems.
- Try the Floral Water Soothing Hydrating Mist on page 121, Acne Face Mask on page 122, Skin Spot Face Serum on page 123, Brightening Face Serum on page 124, and Irritatied/Inflamed Face Serum on page 125.

Cold and flu

Getting colds is super common during pregnancy because your immune system will be weaker than usual. Sometimes they can be harder to shake off because you can't take the supplements you usually take to ward them off. There really isn't a whole lot you can do to eliminate sickness, so prevention is key.

When I was around people who were sick I would take some propolis afterwards. To learn more about the safety of bee products, go to page 13.

Cold and flu prevention:
- Wash your hands often.
- Get some rest. Lots of sleep will keep your immune system strong so take a sick day and curl up in bed. Give yourself permission to take some time off to rest and recuperate.
- Eat foods high in vitamin C like bell peppers, parsley, broccoli, strawberries, cauliflower, and citrus.
- Eat foods rich in zinc like crimini mushrooms, spinach, beef, lamb, and pumpkin seeds.
- Drink ginger or turmeric tea several times a day.
- Drink lots of water. Your baby needs water to create amniotic fluid and you need to stay hydrated to help flush the cold out of your system.
- Make a batch of Homemade Bone Broth on page 107.
- Gargle salt water when you feel an itch in your throat.
- Try taking high quality Echinacea

<u>Nausea</u>

Nausea during the first trimester is very common. The technical term is morning sickness, but nausea can hit any time of the day. For most people, it goes away after the first trimester is over but for others it lasts for the entire pregnancy.

There are a lot of different factors that contribute to morning sickness;
- It can be a way for your body to naturally detox. If you were exposed to a lot of toxins before becoming pregnant, your body is trying to eliminate them in a

hurry, causing lots of liver activity.
- Nausea can also be linked to the hormone changes that go along with pregnancy including the higher estrogen levels.
- Morning sickness that actually happens in the morning can be linked to low blood sugar levels that have dropped overnight. It can also happen when you become too hungry and blood sugar levels drop.
- Strong smells like sweaty subways and foods that are oily or super sweet can cause nausea.
- Dehydration can contribute to morning sickness.
- Lack of exercise, stress, and anxiety may also be the cause of nausea.

For me, the first 6 weeks were pretty much nausea free. I did notice that if I walked my dog before eating breakfast while drinking green tea that I would feel a bit nauseous. I thought this was a sign that I should reduce my caffeine intake, but the culprit was skipping breakfast! I also found I felt nauseous when I had wine with dinner. I didn't know I was pregnant and it was the holiday season so there were lots of celebratory dinners before I found out.

From week 7 onward, I actually felt awesome in the morning but as the day went on I got more and more nauseous. Between 5 pm and 8 pm was the worst for me. I'm lucky because I never actually barfed, but I felt like I was car sick and did a lot of gagging. Thankfully it went away around week 13.

Morning sickness suggestions:
- Vitamin B6 has been found to reduce morning sickness. You can take 25mg 3x per day.
- Acupuncture can be really helpful, just make sure you

tell your acupuncturist that you are expecting.

- Ginger has long been used to reduce nausea. You can drink herbal ginger tea, suck on a pure ginger root, or if that is too strong try ginger candies. I have a great recipe on page 88.
- Drink medicinal teas like Dandelion root tea to support the liver, chamomile tea for its soothing properties, or mint tea to calm the stomach. Drink anise or fennel seed tea in the morning when you wake up.
- Sleep at least 7 hours a night.
- Snack before bed, throughout the night, and before getting out of bed. I liked to keep raw almonds on my bedside table, but unsalted crackers or toast can also work.
- Get out of bed slowly in the morning and avoid any sudden movements.
- Don't take prenatal vitamins on an empty stomach, take them after meals.
- Take 100 mg of magnesium per day.
- Eat before you feel hungry. Nausea usually gets worse when your blood sugar levels drop so if you wait until you feel hungry you might also start feeling nauseous.
- When you are feeling OK, eat nutrient dense foods that are high in protein, healthy fats, and fibre.
- Moderate exercise and working on lowering your stress levels can be really helpful. Exercise will reduce acid and carbon dioxide build up in the blood.
- Drink lots of water throughout the day to avoid dehydration, especially if you are throwing up.
- Go for a walk and get some fresh air; sometimes opening a window can even help.
- Eliminate any strong odors that could trigger nausea and stay away from stinky places.

- Try wearing a nausea bracelet. These can be helpful because they put pressure on the acupuncture point associated with relieving nausea.

Fatigue

Fatigue is a very common symptom in the first trimester because your body is working really hard to support your growing baby and the development of your placenta. It might come back again in the third trimester as the baby's growth accelerates.

I was working a lot during the first trimester so I was pretty tired whenever I wasn't teaching. I got very tired around 2 pm every day. I was lucky enough to squeeze in daily naps, which really helped me stay awake and socialize in the evening if I wasn't feeling too sick. Although on nights that I was super nauseous I would go to bed at 7 pm to avoid the awful feeling.

Fatigue suggestions:
- Get lots of sleep. Try to sleep for at least 8 hours a night and take naps whenever you can. A quick 30 minute nap after work will give you enough energy to get through the evening.
- Take a prenatal vitamin that is high in energy boosting B vitamins.
- Ask your healthcare provider to check your iron levels; low iron is linked to extreme fatigue.
- Reduce stress by asking for help so you can have some time to relax and rest.
- Exercise daily, even if you feel too tired to exercise. A slow walk outside can increase your oxygen intake, improve circulation, appetite, and bowl function. The

sunlight will wake you up and it will reduce stress levels.

Food aversions

Food aversions are really common during the first trimester. The exact cause is unknown, but many doctors believe it is linked to the high levels of human chorionic gonadotropin (HCG). This is the hormone that triggers the positive pregnancy test. It reaches its highest point during the first trimester and tapers off around the 11th week of pregnancy when nausea and food aversion usually start to fade.

I started getting really bad food aversions around week 7. I couldn't stomach meat and even the smell would make me want to throw up! I knew I needed protein but eating meat was just not going to happen during the first trimester. My husband had to cook meat for himself whenever I was out of the house and he made sure to air out the smells before I got home.

The food aversions were really hard for me because I'm someone who lives to eat. I love food! During the first trimester, I would start feeling hungry and think "Oh crap I'm hungry again". I would wish that I could magically fill my stomach with food without having to actually eat anything. The foods I found tolerable were smoothies with protein powder, applesauce with collagen powder and chia seeds, hummus and veggies, and junk food like pizza, fries, cupcakes, and dim sum. I decided that as long as I had a good breakfast when I was feeling OK I would eat whatever seemed appetizing for dinner.

Food aversion suggestions:
- Stick with the food you find tolerable and don't force yourself to eat something that makes you want to gag.
- Sneak protein into your diet using protein powder, chia seeds, and nut butters.
- Try hiding the food you don't want in other foods. If spinach is grossing you out, you might be able to eat it blended in a smoothie because the taste and texture will be hidden.
- Eat the pregnancy power foods, from page 6, when you are not feeling nauseous.

Food cravings

Pregnant ladies are famous for their unusual food cravings that last most of the pregnancy. Cravings may be partially influenced by hormones like estrogen and progesterone, but they can also be a signal that your body is missing a certain nutrient.

I found I randomly craved some foods I hadn't eaten in ages, for example right now I'm really craving hot dogs! I also craved sugary foods a lot during pregnancy which isn't surprising with my history of candida. During my first trimester only certain foods like dim sum, pizza, and fries were appetizing to me.

Food craving suggestions:
- Craving chocolate? Chocolate craving may indicate that you are stressed or feeling down. Chocolate contains magnesium and theobromine which reduce stress levels. When you eat chocolate your feel good chemicals also get a boost. If you are craving chocolate because you are feeling down, take some

time to reflect on what is making you feel this way and reach out to someone you can talk to. Instead of eating chocolate, you can do some stress reduction exercises and look for ways to reduce the stress you are experiencing. Still craving chocolate? Savour a square of high quality dark chocolate or crunch on some raw cacao nibs.

- Carving ice? Ice cravings and other strange cravings for non-food items like dirt and laundry soap are linked to low iron levels. Let your healthcare provider know and ask to have your iron levels tested.
- Craving sugar? Sugar cravings are linked to bacterial overgrowth, lack of sleep, and excessive salt in the diet. If you are craving sweets make sure you sleep 8 hours a night and do not eat too much salty food.
- Craving cheese? Cheese is a well-known comfort food because it contains l-tryptophan, a compound that boosts your mood and promotes relaxation. If you are craving cheese you may need a little TLC. Take some time to yourself to do something you love.
- Craving chips and fried food? These foods are full of unhealthy fats and you crave them when you aren't getting enough healthy fat in your diet. Try eating healthy fats like avocado or coconut oil instead.
- Craving salty foods? Craving salty foods is usually linked to a deficiency in minerals like calcium, magnesium, and zinc. You may want to supplement these minerals or turn to foods that are high in them.
- Craving carbs? Starchy foods like bread, pasta release a feel-good endorphin and serotonin boost. Take some time to figure out what is getting you down and eat some whole grains like quinoa or brown rice.

Mood swings, emotions and stress

With hormones changing, many pregnant women experience mood swings and feel more emotional than they usually do. There can also be a lot of stress during the first trimester as you can get caught up worrying about your baby's health, the symptoms you are experiencing, and the surprise of pregnancy if it was not planned.

I don't think I was overly emotional during the first trimester but I think my husband would disagree. I remember one day I started crying because I came home from teaching and he had organic mac and cheese hot and ready for me to eat and had gone out and bought me cupcakes because I was craving them. I was so overwhelmed by his kindness I started to cry. I also came home from yoga crying one day because I did some deep twisting and learned afterwards that it is not good to do when pregnant.

I was frequently worried and stressed out about my baby's health during the first trimester. It is such a delicate time and I wanted to be doing everything right. It is also hard because unless you have a 7-week ultrasound (which we didn't), you don't really get any sign that the baby is doing well until they can hear the heartbeat around the 10 or 11 week mark. The first time I heard his little heart beating it brought tears to my eyes.

Mood swing, emotions and stress suggestions:
- Try thought shifting – First you need to choose a keyword. It can be "stop", "cancel-cancel", "delete-delete", "nope", something that resonates with you. Whenever you catch yourself worrying about your baby, say the keyword out loud or in your head. When

you say the keyword, it will tell your unconscious
mind not to accept, absorb, keep, or empower any of
these words, thoughts, images, feelings, or sensations.
Instead, it helps you release and let go of the
troubling thoughts.

- Schedule some "me time" to help reduce stress. This
  can be taking 30 minutes in the morning to read a
  book, going for a walk, taking a bath, whatever makes
  you feel relaxed and happy.
- Exercise is a great way to reduce stress. Some great
  activities to do when you are pregnant are prenatal
  yoga, walking, and swimming. You can do any
  exercise you were doing before becoming pregnant as
  long as it feels good. Just make sure you have checked
  with your healthcare provider and teacher to make
  sure it is safe.
- If you are constantly worrying, it might be helpful
  to talk to someone who had a healthy pregnancy.
  They likely experienced the same symptoms that
  are sending you in a worry spiral. It can be very
  reassuring to learn that everything you are feeling is
  totally normal.
- Eat healthy food frequently to stabilize blood sugar
  levels. When blood sugar levels crash you may start to
  feel down or hangry which leads to mood swings.
- Stay hydrated. Dehydration can make you feel
  irritable, tired, and depressed.
- Accept your feeling and fears and talk to someone
  about them. If you are afraid of a certain pregnancy
  complication, talk to your healthcare provider about
  it. It is also important to communicate your fears with
  your partner.
- Give a voice to your emotions by keeping a journal.
  Writing down everything you are feeling can help

release pent up emotions.
- Take a bath using the Soothing Bath Soak on page 112.

Shortness of breath

When you are pregnant your body needs more oxygen. Shortness of breath often happens in the first trimester because your body is producing more of the progesterone hormone. Progesterone increases your lung capacity so you can breathe deeply during pregnancy, however it may take some time to get used to. Shortness of breath can continue throughout the pregnancy as your baby gets bigger and starts to crowd the lungs.

In the first trimester I found I would feel short of breath when exercising. Whenever it happened I needed to take breaks to catch my breath so I wouldn't get dizzy. I also found as my belly got bigger near the end of the second trimester and into the third trimester, it became harder to breathe. I found myself short of breath much more easily.

Shortness of breath suggestions:
- Slowdown and take breaks to catch your breath when you need to. If you are able to lie down it really helps.
- Practice slow deep belly breathing counting at least 4 counts to inhale and 4 counts to exhale.
- I found resting my hands on my head gave me more space to breathe as my belly got bigger.

Sore Boobs

For many people, sore boobs are the first sign of pregnancy. During the first trimester the pregnancy hormones are hard at work preparing your milk ducts so you can feed your baby. For some people this can be an incredibly painful experience but it usually mellows out after the first trimester. Your breasts will grow, your nipple may darken and become larger, and you may get small bumps on your areolas.

My boobs were so sore during the first trimester. When people hugged me I would wince in pain. Shifting in my sleep from one side to another would hurt so much.

Sore boob suggestions:
- Wear a supportive bra that ideally doesn't have underwire. The support will help, but the underwire can cut off circulation to your breasts.
- Sleep in a sports bra.
- Invest in a bra that fits your growing breasts instead of squeezing into the bras that no longer fit.
- As much as possible, avoid anything that will jostle or squish your boobs. This might include running, yoga poses that have you lying on your tummy, sleeping on your tummy, jumping jacks,…
- Take a bath or go swimming. The water will relieve the discomfort and heaviness you might be feeling.

<u>Spotting</u>

About 25% of pregnant women experience spotting or slight bleeding during the first trimester. Although it is terrifying at first, it is usually not cause for concern and there are many things other than miscarriage that can cause it. The fertilized embryo implanting in the uterus around 4 weeks can often cause some spotting. It can also happen because of hormonal changes, after having sex, after doing certain exercises, or after an internal exam.

If you experience any spotting it is always a good idea to call your healthcare provider. They will be able to assess the situation and let you know if there is a cause for concern. Even if you are not concerned, it is still a good idea to let them know.

Spotting suggestions:
- If you are doing yoga or any other form of exercise, make sure you let your instructor know that you are pregnant. It might be strange because you may not have told anyone yet, but it is important to avoid any movements that could disrupt the baby. If your instructor isn't familiar with pregnancy, take some time to do your own research. Some general exercises to avoid are lifting heavy weights, contact sports, horseback riding, hot yoga, and deep twisting.
- Avoid sex, heavy lifting, and any strenuous activity for a few days after spotting has occurred.
- Eat vitamin C rich foods like bell peppers, parsley, broccoli, strawberries, cauliflower, and citrus. Vitamin C can strengthen the blood vessels in the cervix.

Second Trimester

The second trimester is from week 13 to week 26 and it is usually referred to as the golden trimester. Most women stop feeling nauseous around this time and their energy levels start to increase because the placenta is starting to take on a lot of the work.

I loved the second trimester, especially closer to the end when my belly really popped and I started looking pregnant instead of bloated. I had lots of energy, the nausea I was experiencing went away, and I could finally enjoy food again! I also started to feel my baby kicking which was probably my favourite thing about pregnancy.

We did some traveling during the second trimester because I knew it would be uncomfortable later on in the pregnancy. TSA says the body scanners are safe for pregnant women but, the research I have done says they aren't safe for anyone (15). I have always opted for the pat down and usually it only takes a few minutes but I highly recommend allowing lots of extra time just in case. During one of our flights I waited 45 minutes for them to find a female TSA agent to pat me down. I think it would have been even longer if my pregnancy hormones hadn't kicked in and I started crying because I was about to miss my flight. They finally found someone to pat me down and I ended up sprinting to my gate as they were closing it.

The Bump

The second trimester was exciting because my bump popped and was starting to show. It was fun not having to hide it anymore and I loved having people ask me about my pregnancy. I also had fun raiding my friend's closets for maternity clothes. I really didn't want to spend a lot of money on clothes that I would only wear for a few months and I was lucky to have lots of friends who had recently been pregnant. I also found some of my looser shirt still fit during the 2nd trimester.

Favourite things about the 2nd trimester

I loved the amount of energy I had during the second trimester. I didn't feel like I needed to nap anymore and I wasn't falling asleep on the couch at 9 pm. It was nice to bump up our social life a little.

I also started feeling my baby kick around week 16 which was amazing! I was listening to my students present their food demos and all of a sudden there was a little kick that totally threw me off guard. It was so exciting! Whenever I felt something I would get so excited and call my husband over to put his hand on my belly, and then nothing would happen. It took a while for my baby's kicks to be consistent enough for my husband to feel them.

It is such a cool sensation to feel him moving around in there. Even though I could feel the movements internally, I would pretty much always have one hand on my belly. Feeling him kick is really the best thing ever and probably my favourite thing about being pregnant.

Exercise

During the first part of the 2nd trimester my exercise regime stayed the same. I was still walking my dog for 1 or 2 hours a day and going to yoga 3 times a week. Around week 25 the butt muscle pain I was experiencing hit its peak and I had to stop doing yoga and cut down on walks. It took about 3 weeks for the pain to totally go away and I was able to start walking my dog for 2 hours a day again.

Cravings

I didn't have too many cravings during the second trimester. One of the weirder cravings was for hotdogs. I haven't eaten a hotdog in years but I really wanted one! We ended up researching the best hot dogs in Toronto and I thoroughly enjoyed my fancy $10 hotdog. It was not the healthiest lunch but it was delicious.

With the warm summer weather, I also started craving ice cream. One of my favourite things to do is walk along the waterfront with my husband and our dog while enjoying gelato out of a cup. There are some really yummy gelato places that usually have fun dairy-free options. Every now and then I would order a regular dairy based gelato knowing it would give me gas.

Mood

I found I worried a lot less during the second trimester. The anatomy scan and genetic testing came back with no potential problems so I was able to relax. Since I could feel my baby moving around in there, I was no longer worried that something had gone wrong. Those little kicks are so reassuring.

When my butt muscles were really bothering me, I got pretty down. I was in so much pain and I really didn't like the idea of canceling my yoga membership and not exercising. I thought I would be in pain for the rest of my pregnancy and I didn't know how I would deal with that. Thankfully, I was able to use the tips I share in this book to completely eliminate the butt muscle pain.

It is important to remember that nothing is permanent during pregnancy. Everything is changing and growing on a daily basis so something that bothers you now may be totally gone in a week or two.

Sleep

Sleeping in the second trimester was a little more challenging as my belly grew bigger but I was still able to sleep really soundly. I was trying to only sleep on my side and I found having a pillow between my knees was much more comfortable. I also put a pillow behind my back to make sure I didn't sleep totally on my back and to make it easier to roll over. Rolling over with a pillow between your knees really messes up the sheets.

Healthcare

During the second trimester we had monthly visits with our midwives. It was great because we got to know both of the midwives who will be attending the birth along with our student and the alternate midwife. The appointments were a half an hour so we had lots of time to ask any questions we had.

We decided to do a genetic testing ultrasound at 15-weeks and an anatomy scan at 20-weeks so we got to see our baby twice! It was really reassuring to know that everything was looking good.

Near the end of the second trimester the Gestational Diabetes test is usually done. I was not too keen on drinking the liquid that is used for the test because the ingredients are less than stellar. After talking it over with my midwife, we decided it was OK for me to opt-out of this test because my risk factor for Gestational Diabetes was super low.

We also took time during the second trimester to start thinking about our birth preferences. My mom is a hypnobirthing instructor so I knew I wanted to sign up for hypnobirthing classes. We did a lot of research and signed up for a class that started near the beginning of the third trimester.

<u>What I was happy to leave behind</u>

I was SO incredibly happy to leave that butt muscle pain behind! It was so nice when it finally subsided and I was able to move without any pain. I was also really excited to start exercising and doing prenatal yoga again.

I was also happy to leave headaches behind. Around week 15, I started experiencing headaches whenever the weather and pressure changed. It was bad timing since it was spring time and we had lots of rainy days that caused headaches. This lasted for a few weeks and thankfully went away.

The last thing I was happy to leave behind was swelling and

overall puffiness. Around week 25 I noticed that the skin on my calves felt tight when I crouched down and my face looked puffier on TV. After using a bunch of the suggestions in this book, I was able to eliminate the puffiness completely!

Key Supplements

<u>DHA (Docosahexaenoic acid)</u>

DHA is an Omega 3 long-chain fatty acid that is found in the grey matter of the brain and the retina of the eye. Babies in utero cannot produce their own DHA and have to get it from the placenta. DHA is important because it plays a vital role in your baby's brain and eye development.

DHA is found in foods like fatty fish, fish oil, organ meat like liver, and algae. Your body can also convert the omega 3 fatty acids found in walnuts and flax oil into DHA.

<u>Iron</u>

As I mentioned in the first trimester, iron is a significant nutrient during pregnancy. It plays an important role in your baby's brain development including cognitive and behavioural growth.

Absorption rate and the demand for iron rise in the second trimester.

Common discomforts and how to treat them naturally

Abdominal aches

As your body is growing and changing to make room for your growing baby, you will experience lots of aches and pains in your abdomen and groin. This is totally normal and can feel similar to period cramps or like a stitch in your side.

Abdominal ache suggestions:
- Take a warm bath with Epsom salts, not too hot because you don't want to overheat.
- Exercise daily.
- During spasms, take deep relaxing breaths and lean towards the pain to allow the ligaments to relax.

Anemia

During pregnancy your blood volume increases by 50%. Most of this increase is due to additional plasma, which is the liquid part of your blood. Anemia can occur because your plasma is increasing faster than your red blood cells volume. The red blood cells are the ones that carry oxygen to you and your baby's cells.

The symptoms of anemia include fatigue, rapid heartbeat, and pale skin, gums, and eyes. If you find you are craving weird things like coal, dirt, ice, starch, or hair, you might be anemic.

Anemia suggestions:
- Make sure you have enough B vitamins in your diet or

that you are taking a good quality prenatal.
- Eat foods rich in iron listed in the Key Pregnancy Nutrients section on page 2.
- Sea vegetables are an excellent source of iron. Try shaking some dried powdered Dulse or Kombu over your meals; you won't be able to taste it.
- Talk to your healthcare provider about checking your iron levels to determine if you should be taking an iron supplement.
- Cut out caffeine and carbonated drinks because they interfere with iron absorption.
- Cook in cast-iron pans to increase the iron content of your food.

Bladder Infections and UTIs

UTIs are common during pregnancy because of the changes to the urinary tract. As you can probably tell by the more frequent washroom visits, your baby is sitting right on top of your bladder. As your baby gets bigger and heavier, the weight on the bladder can block drainage which can cause infection.

If you think you have a bladder infection or UTI, it is important to get it checked out by your healthcare provider. If left untreated, bladder infections can lead to a kidney infection. Kidney infections may cause early labour or low birth weight.

Bladder infection suggestions:
- Talk to your healthcare provider.
- Wear cotton underwear and avoid tight pants that are not breathable.
- Avoid sugary foods that will feed the bacteria.

- Increase water intake and go pee when you feel the urge. Take time to pee to make sure you have eliminated everything.
- Drink unsweetened cranberry juice – add stevia if you find it too bitter.
- Take probiotics or eat plain yogurt daily.

<u>Bleeding gums</u>

Hormone changes send more blood to your gums which makes them more sensitive and likely to bleed. Bleeding gums happens to about 50% of pregnant women so if your gums are bleeding you are not alone. Once your baby is born, your gums will go back to normal.

Bleeding gums suggestions:
- Use a softer toothbrush and be very gentle when you floss. This is not the time to skip brushing your teeth or flossing all together.
- Try oil pulling with coconut oil, it will clean the bacteria out of your mouth and sooth your gums.
- Make sure your diet contains enough calcium and high quality protein. For a list of foods see the Key Pregnancy Nutrients section on page 2.
- Increase your intake of food rich in vitamin C like bell peppers, parsley, broccoli, strawberries, cauliflower, and citrus.

<u>Body image</u>

It is important to remember that you are growing a baby, not "getting fat".

You will probably be showing by the time the second

trimester comes around but sometimes at the beginning you will just look like you ate a big meal.

Your boobs and belly will be getting bigger for sure, but as your pregnancy progresses you may find your legs, butt, arms, and even your face getting bigger and puffier. These changes can be hard to deal with but it is important to remember that they are all for a good cause. Unless you have been advised to lose weight, it is not the time to diet when you are pregnant.

Body image suggestions:
- Go on a maternity clothes shopping spree and ask around for maternity clothes you can borrow from friends. Dressing up your bump can be really fun so embrace it!
- Go through your closet and pack away any of the clothes that no longer fit. This will make getting dressed much easier and it will force you to stop trying to squeeze into jeans that you can no longer button up. I did this once every trimester and it made getting dressed much more enjoyable.
- Remind yourself that you are not getting fat; you are growing a little human.
- Remember that a lot of the weight you are gaining is for a purpose. Here is an average breakdown: baby is 7.5lbs, placenta is 1lb, amniotic fluid 2lbs, uterus increases by 2.5lbs, boobs increase by 3lbs, extra blood is 4lbs. That totals 20lbs and it doesn't take into account the extra fat that you need for energy. The average woman should gain between 25-35lbs, if you are underweight you need to gain more and if you are overweight you might gain a bit less.
- Create a positive body image affirmation and repeat it daily. You can try "I accept and love my body and the

little baby it is growing".

<u>Congestion and nosebleeds</u>

You can blame hormone changes for increased congestion and nosebleeds you might be experiencing. The hormone changes that occur with pregnancy cause the mucus membranes that line your nose to swell. This makes your nose feel stuffy and can make you snore at night. It can also cause your nose to bleed more easily. If you are having frequent nosebleeds that last over an hour, consult with your healthcare provider.

I have always been prone to nosebleeds so it wasn't a surprise when I started getting them more frequently in the second trimester around week 17. One time I got a nosebleed on the subway between stops and the only thing I had to catch the blood was a tampon, so I stuck it up my nose and hoped no one noticed. It worked so well that I have done it a couple times since then! I have also been known to go to the dog park with toilet paper stuck up my nose because my dog needed to poop and I didn't have time to wait for the bleeding to stop. Pregnancy related nosebleeds didn't last very long which was a relief.

Congestion suggestions:
- Try using a neti pot to gently flush the nasal passage. If you get nosebleeds, just use warm water and no salt.
- Dairy can cause the body to produce excess mucus. Remove dairy from your diet for a week and see if you notice a difference.
- Increase your intake of vitamin C rich foods; like broccoli, cabbage, grapefruit, lemons, oranges,

peppers, and strawberries.

Nosebleed suggestions:
- Moisturise the inside of your nose with coconut oil before going to bed.
- Run a humidifier at night and during the day to keep the air moist.
- Be super gentle when blowing your nose or stop blowing it all together if it starts to bleed every time you blow it.
- If you do get a nosebleed, do not tilt back your head! Look straight ahead, plug your nose and apply pressure to the nostrils to stop the bleeding. You can also roll up some toilet paper or stick a tampon up your nose to catch the blood and help it clot. This is my favourite thing to do because then your hands are free to go about your day. Applying ice to the bridge of your nose can also help with the clotting process.

Gas

Gas is yet another symptom to blame on pregnancy hormones. When you are pregnant, your body has high levels of progesterone. Progesterone is a hormone that relaxes smooth muscle tissue in your body, including your digestive tract. This slows down digestion and can cause gas to build up which leads to bloating, burping, and farting.

Week 23 the farting started for me! I was pregnant during the summer and was constantly craving ice cream. Usually I would go for a dairy free alternative like gelato but every now and then I ordered the real thing. One night after eating at a notoriously delicious ice cream place, I got really bad gas. It didn't hurt or smell, but it was so loud it kept waking me and my husband up all night. It was pretty funny but I learned my lesson, no more dairy filled ice cream!

Gas suggestions:
- Avoid foods that cause gas. Common offenders are beans, and raw cabbage, cauliflower, and broccoli. You can also keep a food diary and track gas for 5 days to help you figure out which foods are causing gas.
- Eat 4-5 small and simple meals a day to ease digestion.
- Eat mindfully and take time to properly chew your food.
- Drink lots of water.
- Exercise daily to prevent constipation and speed up digestion.
- Try taking a digestive enzyme that is safe for pregnant women.

<u>Headaches</u>

During the first trimester, headaches are often caused by the surge of hormones, low blood sugar, hunger, or increase blood volume. If you were someone who drank a lot of coffee and caffeinated drinks before becoming pregnant and decided to quit or cut down during pregnancy, headaches could be due to caffeine withdrawal.

During the second trimester, headaches can be triggered by stress, changes to your vision, dehydration, sinus congestion, or allergies.

Poor posture and lack of sleep can contribute to headaches in the third trimester. If you experience long lasting headaches in the third trimester, it is important to contact your healthcare provider because it could be a sign of preeclampsia.

Around week 15, I started experiencing headaches whenever the weather and pressure changed. It was bad timing since it was spring time and we had lots of rainy days that caused headaches. This lasted for a few weeks and thankfully went away.

Headache suggestions:
- Drink lots of water.
- Take a magnesium supplement.
- Fatigue can cause headaches. Take naps and get at least 7 hours of sleep at night.
- Snack frequently to maintain stable blood sugar levels and to keep you satiated.
- Do neck stretches and relax your jaw to reduce tension related headaches.
- Practice stress reduction techniques like meditation and exercise. Stress causes you to contract muscles which reduces blood flow.
- Try the Headache Blend on page 126.

<u>High Blood Pressure and Preeclampsia</u>

Preeclampsia is very common during pregnancy. The symptoms include high blood pressure, edema, and excess protein in your pee. The cause is actually not known but, if you experience it in a prior pregnancy, you are at increased risk of having it again in following pregnancies. Your healthcare provider will be monitoring your blood pressure on a regular basis to watch for signs of preeclampsia.

High blood pressure and preeclampsia suggestions:
- Essential fatty acids like evening primrose oil can help improve circulation, lower blood pressure, and thin the blood. Consult your healthcare provider before taking this.
- Eating raw garlic can help lower blood pressure.
- Avoid sugar and refined carbohydrates.
- Get lots of rest and sleep.
- Stay hydrated.
- Exercise daily to promote circulation.

Puffiness and Edema

The rise in estrogen during pregnancy encourages the retention of fluids. Many pregnant ladies experience swelling in their feet and legs (hello kankles!) but you can also get puffiness in your arms and face as well. It is important to tell your healthcare provider if you experience any edema because they will want to monitor it. This will continue into the third trimester.

I noticed that my legs were starting to swell around week 25. I would crouch down to pet my dog and wonder why the skin on my calves felt so tight. I also thought my face looked puffier on TV. It actually took me a while to realise it was edema. After using a bunch of the suggestions below, I noticed that it completely went away around week 30.

Puffiness and edema suggestions:
- Stay active and exercise to keep the blood and lymphatic system moving. Walking daily is a great way to exercise.
- When you are sitting down, prop up your legs to encourage blood flow.

- Try not to sit in the same position for too long, switch from standing, to sitting, to lying down as much as possible.
- Water pressure can reduce the discomfort of edema so take a bath or go for a swim.
- Don't limit your water or fluid intake, this will only signal to your body to retain more fluid.
- Reduce salty and processed foods.
- Increase protein intake.
- Wear loose and comfortable clothing to promote circulation. You may even need to get shoes that are half a size larger than usual.
- Only if it feels ok to be on your back, try lying with your legs up the wall.
- Remove any rings you regularly wear, if you wait too long they may have to be cut off!
- Lie on your left side while you sleep to improve circulation.
- Try the Swollen foot rub on page 118 and the Soothing Foot Soak on page 119.

Stretch marks

During pregnancy your belly, butt, boobs, and thighs can grow and expand quickly causing stretch marks. They appear when the skin becomes overstretched and the fibres in deep layers tear. About 90% of women will get stretch marks during the 6th or 7th month of pregnancy, so you are not alone. If your mom has stretch marks, then you are more likely to get them since they can be genetic.

The bad news is that stretch marks don't go away, the good news is that they fade with time and there is a lot you can do to prevent them.

Stretch marks suggestions:

- Massage a nourishing oil or cream to your belly, boobs, butt, and thighs daily. You can start as early as the first trimester so that you are in the habit of doing it daily by the time the second trimester rolls around. Some natural oils and products that work are:
    1. Raw shea butter
    2. A mixture of ½ cup olive oil, ¼ cup aloe vera, liquid vitamin E from 6 capsules, and vitamin A from 4 capsules
    3. Cocoa butter
    4. Sweet almond oil
    5. Coconut oil
    6. Stretch Mark Belly Oil on page 117
- Floral Water Soothing Hydrating Mist on page 121
- Stay hydrated to keep your skin cells plump and more likely to bounce back from the stress caused by stretching.
- Eat a diet rich in skin nourishing foods that are high in vitamin E, vitamin A, and omega 3s. Vitamin E protects the skin cell membranes and can be found in nuts, seeds, avocado, broccoli, and collard greens. Vitamin A repairs skin tissues and can be found in carrots, sweet potatoes, mangos, squash, and red bell peppers. Omega 3 keeps the cell membrane healthy and makes your skin glow. It can be found in fish, walnuts, and eggs.
- Exercise to improve circulation which helps the skin retain its elasticity.
- Try dry brushing. It will exfoliate your skin and increase circulation which keeps your skin healthy. Dry brushing can reduce the appearance of stretch marks you already have and prevent new ones for appearing.

- Collagen improves your skin's elasticity and some believe that taking collagen supplements or drinking bone broth can reduce stretch marks.
- Increase collagen production by eating lots of foods high in vitamin C like broccoli, cabbage, grapefruit, lemons, oranges, peppers, and strawberries.

Third Trimester

The third trimester runs from Week 27 to whenever you give birth. I feel like I got the hang of being pregnant during the third trimester and I started genuinely loving it. I was so excited to meet my baby but I also got sad that my pregnancy journey was almost over. My bump had become a natural extension of my body and I really loved feeling him moving around in there all the time. He was a very active baby!

My baby also started getting hiccups around week 35. I felt bad for him because I know that I don't enjoy having hiccups. Whenever it happened, I tried to take some deep oxygen packed belly breaths to help him out. It always helps me get rid of my hiccups and I think it helped him too.

The Bump

I totally fell head over heels in love with my bump during the third trimester. It really became an extension of my body and I didn't squish it or bang it into things quite as often as I did in the 2nd trimester.

I also had fun dressing up my bump. I enjoyed having a limited wardrobe because it made dressing easier and it allowed me to get creative. I only had a few key things that fit so I found fun ways to accessorise. I was also lucky that is was summer so I wore tons of loose comfy dresses.

My bump did start getting in the way around the 35 week mark. I started spilling food on it because I couldn't get close enough to the table and my plate. It became really hard to put on socks and don't even get me started on shoes! I was really lucky that it was summer time because I lived in my Birkenstocks and didn't wear any shoes that had laces. One day I decided to wear sneakers and my husband had to help me get them on and tie the laces. Putting on underwear, pants, and any bending over also became and challenge.

Favourite things about the 3rd trimester

I loved my bump in the third trimester. It was so big and cute!

My baby was moving almost constantly in the 3rd trimester and I loved it. I spent lots of time having little chats with him. It was a cool way to start connecting with him even though it felt silly at times. Around 35-weeks I also started feeling him get hiccups which were cool.

Exercise

With my butt pain gone I was SO EXCITED to get back on my yoga mat! I decided to go to prenatal classes twice a week. I choose prenatal classes over my regular classes because I was out of shape from the break I took and I wanted to connect with more expecting moms. I loved how each class started with everyone saying their name, how they were feeling, and sharing something else pregnancy related.

I also started swimming once a week for 45 minutes. At 33 weeks my baby was sideways and swimming was a great way to get him into the birthing position. It was also the summer so it was amazing to spend some time outside enjoying the summer.

I continued to walk my dog for 1 or 2 hours a day. My pace was slower but my dog didn't mind. I got a lot of exercise during the third trimester!

Cravings

Nothing is better than in season fruit! I was berry and peach obsessed during the third trimester. When berries were in season, I was literally spending $10 a week on fresh in season berries at the farmer's market. When peaches came into season, I ate a big basket every week, 2-3 peaches a day! I may have gone a bit overboard but they tasted like candy.

I also had a random craving for puffed brown rice cereal with maple syrup and almond milk. It made for a yummy breakfast topped with peaches and some collagen powder for protein.

Mood

My mood was pretty stable throughout my pregnancy. There was one evening around 34 weeks that I started crying like crazy for no reason at all. I just started and couldn't stop. I tried so hard to figure out what was making me emotional but in the end I think it was just hormones. It happened again a few times as the birth of my baby was getting closer. Knowing that my life was going to totally change was really overwhelming and when I'm overwhelmed I cry.

Sleep

Sleep became more difficult for me in the third trimester. It became harder to get comfortable and I found I was restless in the middle of the night. One night I was dreaming that I was doing yoga and getting really deep into pigeon pose. Eventually I woke up and my hips were aching despite all of the pillows I was using to support my pregnant body. And of course I was getting up to go to the washroom 1 or 2 times a night making it harder to get a deep sleep.

I found I started getting tired again during the day. After long walks in the summer heat found that I felt a little fatigued and it would take me a while to cool down and feel normal again. I also started napping almost every day; I figured napping is good training for when the baby comes.

<u>Healthcare</u>

We started going to Hypnobirthing classes at the beginning of the third trimester. I was really focused on having a natural water birth without any pain medication so I knew I needed to do something to prepare. The hypnobirthing philosophy and approach really resonated with me so we decided to sign up for the classes. I loved all of the self-hypnosis techniques we learned and the hypnosis recordings were awesome.

My husband also found the material we covered to be very helpful because and it outlined his role in the birth. After going through the class and practicing leading up to the birth, I was actually looking forward to giving birth and I had absolutely no fear. I also loved listening to the relaxation as I was falling asleep.

My visits to the midwife increased during the third trimester from biweekly to weekly. We also had a few extra ultrasounds because my belly was measuring small. Initially I wanted to keep ultrasounds to a minimum but I figured we were better off safe than sorry. I'm lucky to live in Canada where healthcare is covered so the extra ultrasounds to check on his size and to make sure he was getting the nutrients he needed were at no additional cost to us.

My baby flipped head down week 35 which was a big relief! I was doing everything I could at home to encourage him to flip. I went swimming, spent lots of time with my forearms on the ground and my butt in the air, and did lots of visualization. At one point I got a clear message from my baby asking me to stop nagging him to flip! A few days later we learned he was head down.

<u>What I am happy to leave behind</u>

I was so happy to leave behind having to sleep on my side! I'm usually a back sleeper so being able to sleep on my back, or however I want, will be amazing! I'm looking forward to being able to move gracefully again as well. With an extra 30+ lbs and a big belly, even flipping from my left side to my right side in bed was a bit of an ordeal. Putting on underwear, socks, pants, and shoes was also a struggle that I'm happy to leave behind.

I was also so excited to be able to eat oysters and other foods I had been avoiding for months. I like to eat my meat medium rare and my egg yolks runny so it will be nice to eat them cooked the way I like them again.

Key Supplements

DHA (Docosahexaenoic acid)

DHA is a key supplement during the third trimester. It is a structural fatty acid that is a major building block throughout the body, including the central nervous system, brain, and eyes. It can also help decrease post-partum depression and mom brain.

DHA is found in foods like fatty fish, fish oil, organ meat like liver, and algae. Your body can convert the omega 3 fatty acids found in walnuts and flax oil into DHA. You can also take it as a supplement.

Probiotics

Probiotics can be taken throughout your whole pregnancy but are most important during the third trimester. Probiotics are good bacteria that crowd out the bad bacteria in your gut and throughout your body. They boost your immune system and ensure good digestion. Probiotics can also be used as a preventative treatment for GBS, or Group Beta Streptococcus.

Calcium

Calcium is a bone builder which will help your baby's bones and teeth form, aid in your baby's muscle and heart function, blood clotting, and nerve transmission. It is important in the third trimester because baby's needs for calcium will increase.

Other

Vitamin D and iron are also important to the third trimester. During the third trimester, baby stocks vitamin D stores that will last for the first 2 months of life.

Common discomforts and how to treat them naturally

<u>Back pain</u>

Back pain is very common during pregnancy due to the changes to your body. As your baby bump and boobs grow, your posture and center of gravity will change which can cause back pain. Your body is also producing more progesterone which relaxes your muscles. If you are used to sleeping on your back or stomach, the change in sleeping position can also cause back pain.

I actually found I experienced butt muscle pain rather than back pain, my piriformis muscle was strained due to posture changes. It started around week 16 and came and went until the third trimester, when I decided to take action and do something about it. I also had a chronic mid back injury from years ago start acting up around this time.

I had a fantastic prenatal massage where the massage therapist was able to diagnose the problem and provide me with specific stretches. I also used the tips below to get the pain to pretty much go away.

Back pain suggestions:
- Keep the back flexible with cat and cow by kneeling on all fours and arching and curving your back. Daily gentle stretching can really help.
- Do not stay in one position for too long.
- Pay attention to your posture. Try to engage your lower abs, keep your shoulders back, and align your back as straight as possible. You actually don't want to

be using your butt muscles to tuck in your tail bone.
- Try an underbelly support brace.
- Sleep with lots of padding. Place a pillow between your legs, behind your back, and hug a third pillow to make sure you don't twist. You can also buy a pregnancy pillow.
- Wear shoes with good support and ditch your heels. High heeled shoes will throw off your balance making your posture even more exaggerated. The muscles in your feet are also starting to relax so good support is necessary.
- Use a heating pad or ice pack to encourage circulation to the sore area.
- Take a warm Epsom salt bath. Do not make the bath too hot because you and baby don't want to overheat. You can also try a float tank.
- Swimming is another great way to relieve strain on your back and get some exercise.
- Ask your partner, family member, or a friend to massage your back.
- Try acupuncture, massage, physiotherapy, or visit a chiropractor.
- Switch up your exercise regime. What you are doing could be agitating your back making it worse, so try something new.

Constipation

This can happen around the 9th week of pregnancy due to the increase of progesterone. Progesterone is a hormone that causes the muscle contractions that move food through your intestines to slow down, making it harder to poop. The digestive process slows down so that baby can get as many nutrients as possible. This can make pooping a struggle.

It is also common during the third trimester because baby is taking up so much space in your body and putting pressure on the intestines.

Constipation suggestions:
- Eat lots of fibre to make your poop light, bulky, and easier to pass. You can get it from fruits, veggies, legumes, and seeds. I like to add chia seeds or ground flax seeds to my meals to make sure I'm getting lots and lots of fibre.
- Drink lots of water. Water plays a really important role in the digestive system and dehydration can make your poop heavy and hard to pass. I found drinking water throughout the day, before bed, and throughout the night really helped me have a satisfying morning poop. It did mean more nighttime trips to the bathroom though.
- Add 1 tsp ground flax seeds or chia seeds to water at night and drink first thing in the morning followed by a big glass of water.
- Get daily exercise like walking, swimming, or yoga.
- Place your feet on a stool so you are almost in a squat when you go to the washroom. This will help relax your anal muscles and facilitate pooping. You also don't want to rush while on the toilet, relax and do some deep breathing.
- Consider taking probiotics and magnesium citrate.

<u>Heartburn and acid reflux</u>

Heartburn and acid reflux can be caused by several factors;
- Nervous tension can be a cause because it will disrupt the digestive process.

- Excess stomach acid or too little stomach acid can cause the acid to bubble up the esophagus.
- During pregnancy, hormones are causing your muscles to relax and this also includes the stomach muscles. Lazy stomach muscles can allow stomach acid to move up the esophagus and cause heartburn or acid reflux.
- In the third trimester many of your organs have been displaced to allow room for your growing baby. The stomach gets squished upwards which can cause heartburn or acid reflux.

I experienced acid reflux around the 22-week mark and continued on and off for the duration of my pregnancy. At first, I thought my prenatal vitamin was caught in my throat, but after doing some research I realised it was mild acid reflux. I also experienced heartburn once when eating super spicy food. It was surprisingly painful and my husband was worried I was having a heart attack. I avoided spicy foods for the rest of my pregnancy.

Heartburn and acid reflux suggestions:
- Eat mindfully to signal to your body that you are eating. This will help with overall digestion because you will be in a relaxed state and the body will be able to produce the proper amount of digestive juices necessary. Eating mindfully will also ensure that you properly chew your food and eat more slowly.
- Eat at a table in an upright position and wait at least an hour before lying down after eating. Eating in a slouched position or lying down while you are still digesting will allow digestive juices to travel more easily up the esophagus.
- Avoid heartburn trigger foods like food that are

super spicy, acidic, or fried. Caffeine, fizzy drinks with meals, and dairy can also trigger heartburn.

- Try eating 6 small meals per day instead of 3 big meals.
- Make sure to stay hydrated between meals, but don't drink too much water while you are eating as it can dilute the digestive juices and slow down digestion.
- Chew almonds or try taking 1/4tsp sodium bicarbonate in water. If all else fails, take a Tums, it's not ideal because the ingredients aren't the best but it works in a pinch.
- If you are experiencing acid reflux at night, stop eating 2 hours before bed and sleep with your body propped up.

Hemorrhoids

Hemorrhoids are very common during pregnancy. They are actually varicose veins that occur around your anus. The veins get enlarged due to extra blood flowing through them, increased pressure on them from the uterus, and pushing really hard to poop.

Hemorrhoid suggestions:
- Take a soothing warm bath with Epsom salts.
- Eat lots of fibre and drink lots of water to keep your poop light and bulky. See the section on constipation, on page 79, for more tips to prevent and relieve constipation.
- Drink lots of water, at least ten 8oz glasses per day.
- Place a cold witch hazel compress or lemon juice on your anus to sooth and shrink hemorrhoids.
- Apply baking soda to the area to reduce itching.
- Go for a walk to encourage digestion and elimination.

- Make an herbal sitz bath. Steep 4oz dried witch hazel in ½ gallon of water for 8 hours. Separate the liquid from the herbs and pour into a shallow basin. Sit in the basin for 15 minutes twice a day. Doing this with diluted apple cider vinegar can also help.

<u>Leg cramps</u>

Leg cramps during pregnancy are caused by nutritional deficiencies, electrolyte imbalances, changes to your circulation, and the extra strain on your legs due to the extra weight you have gained.

These are the worst and so annoying! I found I got them most often in my calves when I was sleeping or when I stood on the balls of my feet to reach something in a cupboard.

Leg cramp suggestions:
- Eat foods high in potassium and calcium like almonds, bananas, grapefruit, oranges, salmon, sardines, sesame seeds, tofu, and yogurt.
- While sleeping or sitting, elevate your legs so they are higher than your heart.
- Do not stand in one position for too long, keep shifting your weight from leg to leg.
- Do not point your toes, especially in your sleep or when you wake up. Flexing your feet will help relieve cramps.
- Walk daily to increase circulation.
- Stay well hydrated.
- Take a good quality magnesium and calcium supplement if your healthcare provider feels you aren't getting enough in your food and prenatal vitamin.

- Get a foot and leg massage to promote relaxation, improve circulation, and release any nutrients stored in the muscles.

<u>Varicose veins</u>

When you are pregnant your blood level increases to support your growing baby. That can cause extra pressure on your veins and can lead to spider veins which are the tiny red veins that show up in the third trimester. Pressure on your legs due to your growing baby can also cause surface veins in your legs to become swollen and blue or purple. This can be inherited so ask your mom or grandmother if she experienced varicose veins when pregnant.

I found I saw quite a few spider veins appear on my belly and boobs starting somewhere during the second trimester.

Varicose veins suggestions:
- Keep moving throughout the day to encourage blood flow and circulation. If you sit at a desk for long periods, make a point to get up and walk around every hour.
- If you are sitting for a long period of time at work, prop up your legs. If it feels comfortable you can also lie on your back with your legs up the wall or propped on a chair.
- Try wearing support stockings.
- Get regular exercise to stimulate circulation; walking, and swimming are great options.
- Make sure you are getting adequate amounts of vitamin C. Vitamin C stimulates collagen which will keep your arteries supple. Check out the section on vitamin C on page 29 and consult with

your healthcare provider before taking additional supplements.
- Crossing your legs when sitting can limit circulating and is best avoided.
- Ask your partner or a friend to massage your legs every day to promote circulation.

Recipes

I have included a couple recipes I really enjoyed while I was pregnant. You can find even more healthy and delicious recipes on my website JesseLaneWellness.com and in my cookbooks. Go to page 141 to learn more about my cookbooks and how you can purchase them.

<u>Ginger tea</u>

This tea is the perfect remedy for nausea, it is really easy to make and very soothing. You can enjoy it first thing in the morning on an empty stomach to ease nausea and the maple syrup will boost your blood sugar levels. It is also great late at night or after meals to calm your digestive system. I like to grate my ginger but in a pinch you can just chop it into little pieces.

Prep time: 1 minute | Steeping time: 5 minutes | Serves 1

Ingredients:
- 1 Tbsp fresh ginger, grated and peeled
- 2 cups boiling water
- ½ Tbsp maple syrup
- ½ lemon, juiced

Directions:
1. Place ginger in a big mug. Top with boiling water and steep for at least 5 minutes.
2. Add maple syrup and lemon juice and enjoy hot or let it cool to drink cold.

NOTE: Sometimes ginger can be difficult to grate. I like to freeze my ginger and grate it with a citrus zester.

Homemade Ginger Chews

I ate so many ginger candies in the first trimester that it
started to get expensive! I decided to create my own version
using whole food ingredients like dates for sweetness and
tahini for protein and calcium

Prep time: 5 | Chill time: 2 hours

Ingredients:
- 10 Medjool dates, pitted
- ¼ cup tahini
- 2-4 Tbsp grated ginger

Directions:
1. Place all ingredients in a high-powered blender and
   blend until smooth. You may need to soak the dates
   in water for an hour if you don't have a high-powered
   blender. You can start with 2 Tbsp ginger and add
   more depending on your taste buds.
2. Spoon the mixture into a bread pan lined with wax
   paper, smooth out the top.
3. Place in the freezer to set for 2 hours.
4. Once they have set, remove from the freezer and
   cut into bite-sized pieces or keep in the freezer and
   munch on whenever you feel nauseous.

Blueberry Ginger Smoothie
========================

I love the combination of ginger and blueberries. The blueberries are sweet and the ginger adds a really nice spiciness. This smoothie is a perfect meal replacement for those days that morning sickness is ruining your appetite because it is super easy to drink and contains nausea soothing ginger. I also like to add protein powder to make it more filling and chia seeds for added fibre and blood sugar regulation.

Prep time: 5 minutes | Serves 1

Ingredients:
- 1 cup almond milk
- 1 cup blueberries
- 1 cup spinach
- 1 scoop protein powder
- ¼ thumb ginger or to taste
- 1 Tbsp chia seeds
- 4 ice cubes *if blueberries are fresh and not frozen

Directions:
1. Blend and enjoy!

Breakfast Quinoa

Quinoa for breakfast?!?! Why not! If you add the right ingredients quinoa is a great alternative to your morning oats. Breakfast Quinoa is a wonderful protein packed breakfast that will keep you feeling full for hours. Whole grains like quinoa are generally rich in B-vitamins which are essential during pregnancy because they help with baby's brain and nervous system development and they will keep your energy levels high.

Prep time: 5 minutes | Cook time: 15 minutes | Serving size: 2 large servings

Ingredients:
- 2 cups almond milk
- 1/4 Tbsp cinnamon
- 1/2 tsp vanilla
- Pinch ground cloves
- Pinch ground nutmeg
- Pinch ground ginger
- 1 cup uncooked quinoa
- 1/2 cup dried cranberries, or any dried fruit
- 1 Tbsp maple syrup
- 1/2 cup raw almonds, chopped
- 2 Tbsp raw sunflower seeds
- 1 cup fresh blueberries or any fresh fruit
- 2 Tbsp cup chia seeds
- Coconut milk for drizzling

Directions:
1. Mix almond milk, cinnamon, vanilla, cloves, nutmeg and ginger in a pot then add the quinoa. Bring to

a boil, cover and lower the heat to simmer for 10 minutes. Remove from heat and let sit for 5 minutes.

2. Stir in the dried cranberries and maple syrup and adjust sweetness to taste.

3. Spoon the quinoa into bowls and top each serving with almonds, sunflower seeds, blueberries, chia seeds and a drizzle of coconut milk and enjoy!

Carrot Molasses Muffins

Carrot Molasses Muffins are super moist and taste like gingerbread. They are made with nutty spelt flour, sweetened with iron rich blackstrap molasses and laced with nausea soothing ginger. With all of the extra blood circulating your body, iron is super important.

Prep time: 15 minutes | Inactive prep time: 5 minutes | Cook time: 30 minutes | Serving size: 12 medium muffins

Ingredients:
- 2 cups spelt flour
- ¼ cup walnuts, ground
- 1 tsp baking soda
- 1/2 tsp Himalayan rock salt
- 3/4 tsp ground ginger
- 1/2 cup blackstrap molasses
- 1/3 cup coconut oil, melted
- 1/2 cup almond milk
- 2 Tbsp ground chia seeds, 6 Tbsp water
- 1/2 tsp vanilla
- 1 cup grated carrots

Directions:
1. Preheat oven to 350F and line a muffin tin with liners or grease with coconut oil.
2. Grind chia seeds and add water. Mix and set aside to gel for 5 minutes.
3. Mix spelt flour, ground walnuts, baking soda, salt and ginger together in a large bowl.
4. In a small bowl mix blackstrap molasses, melted coconut oil, almond milk, chia eggs and vanilla.
5. Add the wet mixture to the dry mixture and mix until

incorporated.

6. Fold in the carrot pulp until just mixed.

7. Spoon the muffin mixture into the muffin tin until ¾ full and bake for 30 minutes or until a toothpick inserted in the center comes out clean.

Green Eggs

Eggs are a protein powerhouse which is so important during pregnancy because your baby's cells are growing like crazy and protein is the main building block for those cells. Some pregnant women have trouble eating greens during the first trimester so it can help to puree them into eggs.

Prep time: 5 minutes | Cook time: 5 minutes | Serving size: 2

Ingredients:
- ½ cup packed basil
- ½ cup packed spinach
- ½ Tbsp organic butter
- 4 organic eggs
- Salt and black pepper to taste

Directions:
1. Very finely chop the basil and spinach. Do this in a small food processor or by hand, the smaller the pieces the greener the healthy scrambled eggs will look.
2. Place organic butter in a skillet over medium low heat.
3. Crack 4 eggs into a bowl, add the basil and spinach and whisk until mixed.
4. Pour the eggs into the skillet and gently pull the eggs to the center of the pan letting the liquid run to the sides. Keep continually moving the eggs until they are just set (no longer liquid but still shiny), 2-4 minutes.
5. Season with salt and black pepper to taste and serve hot with sprouted bread.

<u>Gluten-free Quiche</u>

Gluten-free Quiche is a great grab and go snack or meal that will keep you feeling full. It is high in protein due to the eggs and the almond flour crust. Eggs are high in choline, which promotes baby's overall growth and brain health so they are a great addition to your pregnancy diet.

Prep time: 30 minutes | Cook time: 1 hour | Serving size: 1 dozen

Ingredients:
Crust

- 2 cups almond flour
- ½ tsp salt
- ¾ tsp baking soda
- ¾ cup melted coconut oil
- 1.5 Tbsp water

Filling

- ½ red onion, finely diced
- 2 garlic cloves
- 2 handfuls of baby spinach, chopped
- ½ cup sun-dried tomatoes, sliced
- ½ cup red olives, pitted and sliced
- 4 organic eggs
- ¼ cup nutritional yeast
- 2 Tbsp almond milk
- Pepper to taste

Directions:
1. Preheat the oven to 350F and line a muffin tin with muffin liners.

2. For the crust, whisk together the almond flour, salt, and baking soda. Add ½ cup melted coconut oil and 1.5 Tbsp water, adding more oil as needed until mixture comes together. The pastry crust should be crumbly but hold together when pressed into a ball.

3. Press the pastry crust into the muffin liners covering the bottom and halfway up the sides. The gluten-free quiche crust should be roughly half a centimeter thick. Poke a couple holes in the bottom of each quiche with a fork and place in the oven for 10 – 15 minutes, until lightly brown.

4. While the crust is cooking, sauté the onions in a frying pan over medium heat for 5 minutes.

5. Add the garlic and sauté until fragrant, roughly 2 minutes.

6. Add the baby spinach and sauté until wilted, roughly 5 minutes.

7. Turn off the heat and stir in the sun-dried tomatoes and olives and set aside.

8. In a medium sized bowl beat the eggs with the nutritional yeast, milk, and pepper until frothy.

9. Once the crust is golden brown, remove from the oven and spoon the filling mixture into the crust. Top with the egg mixture and use the back of a spoon to smooth the top.

10. Place the quiches into the oven and bake until the eggs have set, roughly 20-40 minutes.

<u>Hummus</u>

I love hummus! When I was in Israel the hummus was so good I literally ate it with a spoon. While I was pregnant I was a total hummus monster. During the first trimester I ate a lot of carrots, celery or cucumber dipped in hummus. If you are pressed for time you can always buy hummus but it is pretty quick to make at home if you have a food processor.

Prep time: 10 minutes | Serving size: 2 cups

Ingredients:
- 2 garlic cloves
- 2 cups cooked chickpeas (19oz drained and rinsed)
- 1 lemon, juiced
- ¼ cup tahini
- 2 Tbsp olive oil
- ½ Tbsp cumin
- ½ tsp cayenne pepper
- ¼ tsp black pepper
- Salt to taste

Directions:
1. Place the garlic in a food processor and process until chopped.
2. Add the chickpeas, lemon juice, tahini, olive oil, cumin, cayenne pepper, black pepper and salt and blend until smooth.
3. Enjoy with crackers, carrots, celery, cucumber, tomatoes, peppers, or any of your favourite veggies.

<u>Crispy Chickpeas</u>

Getting enough protein is really important during the first trimester so I was always looking for protein packed snacks. Crispy chickpeas were one of my favourites because not only are they high in protein and fibre but they help curb cravings for chips. They have a crunchy texture and just enough salt to squash your cravings without causing an imbalance.

Prep time: 5 minutes | Cook time: 45 minutes | Serving size: 2 cups
Ingredients:
- 2 cups cooked chickpeas, patted dry
- 3 Tbsp coconut oil, melted
- 1 tsp sea salt
- ½ tsp garlic powder

Directions:
1. Toss the chickpeas with the coconut oil, garlic powder and salt.
2. Place on the baking sheet and bake for 25-45 minutes, mixing every 15 minutes, until crunchy.
3. Enjoy as a fibre and protein packed snack or on top of a caesar salad.

<u>Superfood Trail Mix</u>

Superfood Trail Mix contains a highly nourishing mix of nuts and superfoods that provide you with an excellent source of omega-3s which is great for you and your baby's brain health. It is also high in fibre and protein which are both important for pregnancy.

Prep time: 5 minutes | Serving size: 3 cups

Ingredients:
- 1 cup almonds
- 1 cup walnuts
- 1 cup dried superfoods – I used black mulberries, golden berries, and raw cacao nibs.

Directions:
1. Place everything in a mason jar and shake to mix.

<u>Egg-Free Caesar Salad</u>

I love Caesar salad and I really missed it when I was pregnant because the dressing usually contains a raw egg. I decided that I instead of missing it, I would create my own egg-free Caesar salad dressing. This Caesar Salad has a creamy, egg-free dressing that is much tastier than the bottled version. I also left out the anchovies because I think the smell would make most pregnant women nauseous.

I like to top it with crunchy chickpea croutons which are a protein packed gluten-free substitute for bread croutons. If you follow a vegan or vegetarian diet, you can simply leave out the chicken!

Prep time: 20 minutes | Cook time: 15 minutes | Serving size: 2 mains or 4 sides

Ingredients:
- 2 chicken breasts *omit of vegan/vegetarian
- 2 heads of romaine lettuce, chopped or torn into bite size pieces
- 4 Tbsp nutritional yeast* optional

Dairy Free Caesar Dressing:
- 1 garlic clove
- 2 Tbsp tahini
- 3 Tbsp apple cider vinegar
- 1 Tbsp lemon juice (1/4 lemon)
- 3 Tbsp water
- 1 tsp Dijon mustard
- ½ avocado
- ¼ tsp black pepper
- 1.5 Tbsp capers

Directions:
1. Place the chicken in a frying pan and fill with enough water to cover half of the chicken. Bring the water to a boil, lower the heat and simmer covered for 15 minutes, turning halfway. Once the chicken is cooked let it cool and then cut into 2cm cubes.
2. Make the dressing by mincing the garlic clove in a food processor. Add the remaining ingredients and pulse until smooth. Add additional water if the dressing is too thick.
3. To assemble the salad, place the lettuce in a bowl and toss with the dressing. Top the salad with the diced chicken breast, crispy chickpeas (page 99) and a sprinkle of nutritional yeast.

<u>Bean Salad</u>

I love beans for pregnancy because they are high in fibre and protein. When you are pregnant your digestive system slows down and many women experience constipation and hemorrhoids. Eating high fibre foods is a great way to keep things moving well. Beans are also high in important pregnancy nutrients like iron, folate, calcium, and zinc.

Prep time: 20 minutes | Cook time: 15 minutes | Serving size: 4

Ingredients:
- 1 cup quinoa, uncooked
- ½ cup green olives
- ½ cucumber
- 1 cup cherry tomatoes, quartered
- ½ cup roasted red pepper
- 1 cup edamame
- ¼ cup pine nuts
- 15 oz can kidney beans, drained and rinsed

Dressing
- ¼ cup apple cider vinegar
- ¼ cup olive oil
- 2 Tbsp maple syrup
- 1 Tbsp tamari

Directions:
1. Cook quinoa as directed on the package and set aside to cool.
2. Whisk together dressing ingredients and set aside.
3. Once the quinoa has cooled, place it in a large bowl with the remaining salad ingredients.

4. Pour the dressing over the salad and toss to coat.

Mediterranean Quinoa Salad

Mediterranean Quinoa Salad makes a refreshing vegetarian side dish or main event. The roasted red peppers are bursting with flavour and are complemented by the cilantro and green onions. Whole grains like quinoa are great to enjoy during pregnancy because they are packed with fibre and vitamins. Fibre is important during pregnancy because your digestive system can get sluggish, which leads to constipation. Fibre is a great way to keep everything moving smoothly.

Prep time: 20 minutes | Cook time: 20 minutes | Serving size: 4

Ingredients:
- 1 red pepper
- 1 cup uncooked quinoa
- 2 Tbsp extra virgin olive oil
- Juice of one lime
- 1 tsp ground cumin
- Salt and pepper to taste
- 1/2 cup cilantro, chopped
- 3 green onions, chopped
- 1 Tbsp chia seeds
- 1/2 cup black olives, chopped (optional)

Directions:
1. If you are roasting the red pepper, pre-heat the oven to 400F. Wash the red pepper and place it whole on a baking sheet. Bake for 20 minutes turning every 5 minutes until all of the sides are darker in color. Remove from the oven and let cool for 10 minutes. When the pepper is cool enough to touch, peel

off the skin and remove the seeds. Dice into 1 cm
squares.

2. Cook quinoa as directed on the package. When the
    quinoa is cooked set it aside to cool.

3. In a large bowl combine olive oil, lime, cumin, salt
    and pepper. Whisk until mixed. Add the cilantro,
    green onions, chia seeds, black olives and red pepper
    and toss.

4. Finally add the quinoa, toss until mixed and serve the
    salad at room temperature or place in the fridge to
    serve chilled.

<u>Homemade Bone Broth</u>

Animal bones are a great source of collagen which can help reduce stretch marks. Since we can't digest animal bones, by simmering the bones for a long time, it breaks down the protein into a gelatin which we can digest. If you are experiencing nausea and having a hard time eating, bone broth is a great way to get some nutrients into your body and to keep you hydrated.

Prep Time: 20 minutes | Cook Time: 1 hour + 12-24 hours

Ingredients:
- 3-4 lbs of mixed organic beef bones
- 2 medium carrots, chopped
- 3 celery stalks, chopped
- 2 medium onions, chopped
- 1 Tbsp of coconut oil
- 2 Tbsp apple cider vinegar
- 1 bay leaf
- Water

Directions:
1. Preheat oven to 400F. Place bones in a single layer on a sheet or roasting pan. Drizzle with coconut oil to evenly coat.
2. Roast for 30 minutes, then, flip each bone over and roast for an additional 30 minutes.
3. In a large crock pot or soup pot put the roasted bones, chopped vegetables, bay leaf, and cider vinegar. Cover completely with water and bring to a high simmer.
4. Reduce the heat to low and let simmer for 12-24

hours. Throughout simmering, add water as needed to keep all the ingredients submerged. Once the homemade bone broth has reached a dark rich brown colour, remove from heat.

5. Discard the bones, vegetables, and bay leaf. If you like a smooth broth you can strain through a cheesecloth or nut milk bag.

6. Cool the pot to room temperature then pour into jars. Cool in the refrigerator for at least 1 hour.

7. Before serving, skim the condensed fat off the top of the broth and heat to the desired temperature or enjoy cold.

Kale Oregano Pesto Salmon

Kale Oregano Pesto Salmon is a delicious and easy way to dress up your salmon. Salmon is really high in omega-3 fatty acids which are essential during pregnancy. Omega-3s help build baby's brain and eyes. What sets this recipe apart from the rest is the kale oregano pesto which is a fun and flavorful play on traditional pesto.

Prep time: 10 minutes | Cook time: 20 minutes | Serving size: 2-4

Ingredients:
- 3 garlic cloves
- ½ cup olive oil
- 4 cups of kale, stems removed and roughly chopped or torn
- ¼ cup fresh oregano, stems removed
- ¼ cup sunflower seeds
- ¼ cup nutritional yeast
- 2 large filets of wild salmon
- Salt and pepper

Directions:
1. Preheat the oven to 400F.
2. Place the garlic in a food processor and pulse until minced. Add the olive oil, kale and oregano and pulse until finely chopped. Finally add the sunflower seeds and nutritional yeast and pulse until mixed.
3. Check salmon for bones, rinse under cold water then pat dry. Season both sides of the salmon with salt and pepper.
4. Place each salmon filet on a square of parchment paper and spread 1cm thick layer of pesto on top.

Fold the parchment paper around the salmon creating a pouch. Seal the top by folding it over and twist the ends to create a seal.

5. Bake for 20 minutes or until the salmon is cooked through and flaky. Use the leftover pesto to flavor a side of broccoli, asparagus, kale or any vibrant cooked green.

Aromatherapy, Essential Oils, and Pregnancy

I have always been a big fan of essential oils! They are a great way to naturally add scent to homemade beauty products, they work wonders on skin related issues, they are great for cleaning, and I love diffusing them to naturally scent the air. I love using my various roll-ons to help cure headaches, acne, and calm the nervous system.

When I became pregnant I did a quick search and discovered that not all essential oils are safe for pregnancy. Since I'm not an expert in the field, I asked my friend Andrea Ashley to help me out. She is has an education in advanced skincare, master clinical aromatherapy, diplomas in both organic skincare science and organic skincare formulation and certifications in holistic therapies. You can learn more about Andrea Ashley in the guest author section on page 139.

It is really important to always talk to your healthcare provider before using ANY essential oils when pregnant.

Essential Oil Safety

As much as essential oils have become trendy and easily accessible, it does not mean that you can be using them without caution or knowledge. Each oil is completely unique and so complex that it is truly important to know and understand what you are working with and why. Now, this is not meant to cause may alarm or scare you from using essential oils, because in my opinion they are still safer than pharmaceuticals to use, but rather just to educate you and to keep you and your baby safe.

Many people wonder if it is safe to use essential oils with pregnancy, and the answer is not clear cut. Many certified and experienced aromatherapists have varying answers to that question each with a justifiable reasoning that are worth taking in to consideration. However, my answer is first and foremost always to be safe. Every one of us has different health concerns and pregnancy risks that are best discussed with your certified aromatherapist if you want to be using this modality as treatments during your pregnancy.

There are several ways to use essential oils; topically (through external application on the skin), inhalation (via diffusing or aroma steam), and for some very few oils internally through an experienced aromatherapist using safe methods, dosages, and specific types of essential oils. However, from my personal experience I would never recommend anyone taking any essential oil internally. Food grade or not does not necessarily make ingesting an essential oil safe or effective, nor is it necessary to achieve the beautiful health properties many of you are seeking.

<u>Essential oils to avoid</u>

When discussing the following oils to avoid while pregnant, it is important to avoid the oils altogether as they can be absorbed into your system regardless of the method used.

To address safety, here are some commonly available oils that are best avoided during pregnancy and breast feeding (16):
- Anise
- Basil
- Carrot seed
- Clary Sage
- Cinnamon
- Cypress
- Dill
- Fennel
- Geranium
- Lemon balm
- Lemon verbena
- Lemongrass
- Melissa
- Myrrh
- Sage
- Tea tree
- Thyme
- Wintergreen
- Spanish lavender due to the high camphor content

While this is comprehensive list of essential oils to "not use during pregnancy" it does not necessarily clear all other readily available essential oils and dccm thcm safc throughout your nine months. Through my years of education and experience in Aromatherapy, I have also discovered there are a few other oils that could potentially be added to that list and worth understanding before usage:

- Rose essential oil is a gentle emmenagogue (stimulates menstruation), cleansing, purifying, regulating the female sexual organs and regulating menstrual functions. Avoid using Rose during pregnancy in external aromatherapy applications. Use rose hydrosol instead.
- Oregano is a powerful emmanagogue and is not to be used during pregnancy.
- Atlas Cedarwood essential oil is an abortifacient and best avoided during pregnancy.
- Frankincense is also an emmanagogue. It is advisable to avoid during the first trimester of pregnancy.
- Jasmine is said to not for use by nursing mothers as there have been some findings on Jasmine inhibiting lactation.
- Ylang Ylang can have a balancing effect on hormones and offer hormonal support, best to avoid use during pregnancy.
- Clary sage essential oil is estrogen-like compounds that is best not to be used in aromatherapy treatments when pregnant.
- Nutmeg contains a compound called myristicin that has been shown to cross the placenta causing an increase in the foetal heartbeat.

Now that all of the potential risks have been presented to you it really comes down to you to proceed with common sense and reason. While some essential oils may have a potential risk as we outlined above, do they really compare to the risk associated with conventional drugs should you need to fight an infection or illness during pregnancy?

Kurt Schnaubelt gives an excellent example of this explaining, "say a pregnant women contracts bronchitis of the lower respiratory tract. Should she choose the appropriate use of oregano oils, despite the fact some books recommend against it, or should she turn to the traditional medicine for her condition with a round of hard-hitting, immune-supressing and otherwise unpredictable antibiotics?" And even continues on to say "But, if specific or more severe conditions necessitated, one could arrive at the conclusion that even more forceful use of essential oils might still be a much more reasonable approach then allopathic drugging." (17).

And I have to say, I agree. In saying this, here are a few very basic DIY recipe examples outlining beneficial ingredients to use pertaining to some common pregnancy complaints.

DIY Essential Oil Recipes

These recipes are for informational purposes only. Always check with you certified aromatherapist or healthcare provider before using specific oils or DIY recipes during your pregnancy. For any DIY recipes, always perform a patch test first on your forearm to ensure these ingredients are OK for you.

Stretch Mark Belly Oil

This is the perfect recipe to prevent stretch marks! Vitamin E can help combat stretch marks by promoting skin elasticity. When your skin is more elastic it is much more tolerable to being stretched and therefore minimizes damage. Avocado oil contains a combo of good fatty acids and high concentrations of Vitamin A, E, and D which improves skin elasticity. Coconut oil helps soften skin and has been claimed to reverse damage. Cocoa butter is known to firm, tone and hydrate skin. Lavender essential oil is a general tonic for all skin types and a powerful skin regenerator.

Ingredients:
- 20g Cocoa Butter
- 40g Coconut Oil
- 20g Avocado Oil
- 5g rosehip seed oil
- 5g Vitamin E
- 1g of Lavender Essential Oil

Directions:
1. Double boil cocoa butter to bring to a liquid. You can adjust consistency by adding more cocoa butter to customize to your preference.
2. Turn off heat and add the coconut oil.
3. Once heat is reduced add in avocado oil, followed by rosehip seed oil, vitamin E and lavender essential oil.
4. Mix thoroughly.
5. Use as desired. Best benefits come from daily use, morning and evening.

Swollen Foot Rub

Shea Butter has been used by Native healers for muscle aches and strains, arthritis, and skin treatments (18), making this a wonderful addition to the Soothing Swollen Foot Rub. Pomegranate has contains punicic acid which is anti-inflammatory- perfect for sore swollen feet. Argan oil also considered an anti-inflammatory. Chamomile essential oil is great for swelling and inflammation.

Ingredients:
- 70g Shea Butter
- 20g Pomegranate Oil
- 10g Argan Oil
- 1g Chamomile Essential Oil

Directions:
1. Hand mix ingredients until thoroughly combined. You can adjust consistency by adding more shea butter to make it thicker or reducing the shea butter to make it thinner to customize to your preference.
2. Use as desired.

<u>Soothing Foot Soak</u>

If you find yourself on your feet for long periods of time, this foot soak will feel awesome. Himalayan salt is rich in over 80 trace minerals and is said to be great for healing and detoxifying. Chamomile hydrosol is soothing.

Ingredients:
- ¼ cup of Himalayan Salt
- 60 ml Chamomile Hydrosol
- Warm water

Directions:
1. Fill a foot bath with warm water and add your ingredients and mix thoroughly.
2. Soak for 20 minutes.

<u>Soothing Bath Soak</u>

This bath soak has so many benefits! Is it anti-inflammatory, disinfectant , anti-bacterial (great for acneic skin), skin softening, skin moisturizing, healing of skin conditions of all kinds, and calming to nervous system.

Ingredients:
- ¼ cup of honey
- 10 ml avocado oil
- 10 drops of Lavender essential oil

Direcitons:
1. Mix lavender essential oil with avocado oil to properly dilute and disperse the essential oil.
2. Add oil mixture to honey and mix thoroughly.
3. Draw a warm bath, slowly pouring honey mixture into water and dispersing with hands.
4. *Another option is while in the bath take some on the mixture into your hands and massage it into the skin to get an even more deep hydrating treatment

<u>Floral Water Soothing Hydrating Mist</u>

Hydrosols is a by-product from the distillation of essential oils. In most cases hydrosols are very friendly to the skin, being mildly antiseptic, astringent, and lightly fragrant. It is a great alternative to essential oils when working with children or pregnant women. Chamomile hydrosol is hydrating and soothing. Rose hydrosol is very gentle and provides subtle soothing properties to support hydration of the skin. It is safe for all skin types and babies. Both Roman Chamomile and Rose hydrosol are also great for stretch marks, so this can double as a hydrating body spritz as necessary.

Ingredients:
- 20 ml of Lavender Hydrosol
- 40 ml of Roman Chamomile hydrosol
- 40 ml of Rose Hydrosol

Directions:
1. Pour all hydrosol in a 100ml glass bottle with spray nozzle and gently mix.
2. Use to cool and hydrate the skin as necessary.

Acne Face Mask

While we cannot necessarily treat the underlying cause of the acne as it may be hormonal with an onset during pregnancy, we can treat the symptoms by soothing and cleaning the skin to improve the condition as best as possible. Lemon essential oil has astringent properties. Chamomile essential oil is great for reducing inflammation, acne, blemished skin, psoriasis, and swelling. Bentonite Clay will remove impurities and stimulate circulation to the area treated.

Ingredients:
- 30 g Bentonite Clay
- Filtered Water or Lavender Hydrosol as needed
- 2 drops Lemon Essential Oil
- 2 drops Chamomile Essential Oil

Directions:
1. Pour 30g of clay into bowl. You can adjust consistency by adding more clay to make it thicker or reducing the clay to make it thinner to customize to your preference.
2. Slowly add water or hydrosol while mixing in with clay until you form a smooth paste. If you have sensitive or dry skin, replace water with honey instead to make it less intense.
3. Add 2 drops of chamomile essential oil, 2 drops of lemon essential oil and mix until thoroughly combined.
4. Apply to skin for 10 minutes (it will dry and get flaky!).
5. Rinse with water, pat dry.

Skin Spots Face Serum

Avocado oil contains Vitamin A, B and E as well as amino acids. Avocado oil can help support and prevent aging and damaged skin as well as minimize sun damage. Castor oil has been said help with age spots. Rosehip oil aids in regeneration of skin cells.

Ingredients:
- 8g Avocado Oil
- 2g Rosehip Seed Oil
- 1g Castor Oil

Directions:
1. Mix ingredients until thoroughly combined.
2. Pour into a 15ml glass bottle with pump top.
3. Use as desired after cleansing the skin.

<u>Brightening Face Serum</u>

Jojoba is moisturizing and beautifully compatible with our skin. It is emollient, regenerative and toning (18). Rosehip is nourishing and filled with vitamins, minerals and lycopene (18). Sea Buckthorn has the ability to promote regeneration of skin cells, high in vitamin A carotenes, vitamin E, C and flavonoids as well as essential fatty acids. Rosemary essential oil is stimulating and is great for sluggish skin.

Ingredients:
- 8g Jojoba Oil
- 3g Rosehip Seed Oil
- 2g Sea Buckthorn
- 0.8g Rosemary Essential Oil

Directions:
1. In a small glass dish measure thoroughly mix all of the ingredients.
2. Pour into a 15ml glass bottle with pump.
3. Apply in evening after cleansing.

<u>Irritated/Inflamed Face Serum</u>

Sweet almond oil is rich in proteins, fatty acids and vitamins including, A, B, and E as well as oleic and linoleic essential fatty acids. It is great for irritated skin. Calendula oil contains anti-inflammatory properties. Chamomile and lavender essential oils are both great for soothing irritated and inflamed skin.

Ingredients
- 9g Sweet Almond Oil
- 5g Calendula Oil
- 0.1g Lavender Essential Oil
- 0.1g Chamomile Essential Oil

Directions:
1. Thoroughly mix all of the oils in a small glass dish.
2. Pour into a 15ml glass bottle with pump.
3. Apply as desired after cleansing.

<u>Headache Blend</u>

Diffusing a few drops of lavender and/or chamomile can be helpful. They are not the strongest essential oils for headache relief such as peppermint and rosemary can be, but a great calming alternative.

<u>Yoga and Pregnancy</u>

Before becoming pregnant I was going to yoga 3-4 times a week and I hoped to continue that throughout my pregnancy to keep back pain at bay and to keep me feeling calm and grounded.

I was able to continue with my regular yoga classes up until the end of the second trimester. I really had to listen to my body and make lots of modifications. It was a great exercise of leaving my ego at the door. There were so many poses like fun arm balances I no longer felt comfortable doing and I had to use props when normally I wouldn't. Sometimes I was doing something totally different from everyone in the class and I had to learn to be OK with that.

Around week 25 I found that yoga was actually contributing to the butt muscle pain I was experiencing. I actually cried (thank you pregnancy hormones) when I had to cancel my monthly yoga pass. I took a few weeks away from yoga to give my piriformis time to heal then started going to prenatal yoga classes.

I'm so passionate about yoga I really wanted to include a section about it in this book. Since I'm not an expert in the field, I asked my mom to help me out. My mom, Margot Schelew, is a yoga teacher with prenatal training, a hypnotherapist, and a hypnobirthing instructor.

You can learn more about her in the guest author section, on page 137, and on her website at hypnosisinthecity.ca

Benefits of prenatal yoga

Through the practice of yoga and meditation, you will improve your focus, learn to relax during labour, as well as how to cope with any stress that arises, whether during pregnancy or after the baby is born. There are a lot of fears and worries that pregnant women deal with. Yoga, paired with a cardiovascular exercise such as walking or swimming, can be an ideal way to stay in shape during pregnancy. Yoga keeps you flexible, tones the muscles, and improves balance and circulation, with little impact on the joints.

Yoga is also beneficial because it helps you learn to breathe deeply and relax, which will come in handy as you face the physical demands of labour, birth, and motherhood. One of the first things you learn in a yoga class is how to breathe fully. This breathing calms both mind and body, providing the physical and emotional stress relief the body needs throughout the experience of pregnancy. Taking a prenatal yoga class is also a great way to meet other moms-to-be and embark on this journey together.

<u>Reduces low back pain & sciatica</u>

When you become aware of proper body alignment, you can carry yourself and your extended belly in an integrated manner. This can help to reduce the degree of pelvic tilt associated with pregnancy and significantly reduce the lower back pain which it can cause. As well there are specific yoga poses which target the muscles and tissues associated with the lower back, hips, and hamstrings.

Reduces swelling & inflammation around the joints

Doing yoga regularly improves circulation of blood and oxygen throughout the body, which in turn can reduce swelling and inflammation around ankles and wrists.

Aids in digestion

As baby grows, the intestinal organs get pushed around, which may affect your regularity and cause indigestion. Safe and gentle rotations and forward folds can help to promote regularity and aid in overall digestive flow.

Helps prepare a mother-to-be physically for giving birth

A regular practice of the squatting asana helps to tone muscles of the pelvic floor and helps you gain the strength to remain comfortable in a squatting position. This is an integral part of any yoga program as it helps to familiarize you with these very useful muscles. Even if you choose not to squat during labour, you will want to be able to use these muscles efficiently and effectively when nature calls upon you to push your baby into the world. Couple this with the ujjayi breath and you have the tools you need in the delivery room. You can learn to breathe in a way that is relaxing and natural. When a student consistently practices moving through the asanas in unison with their breath, they will have great familiarity with this powerful relaxation and pain management tool. As well, many yoga poses can translate wonderfully into comfortable labouring positions.

When it comes time to ride through the most powerful of contractions, visual imagery combined with breath work can be one of the most useful labour tools. The weeks of squatting were not done in vain! Squatting combined with a kegel-like movement during pregnancy can really help labour in two ways. If an epidural is done, the loss of sensation in the pelvic floor could make pushing the baby out a bit of a guessing game. If the mom-to-be is used to working with these muscles, they will find it easier to use them even if they cannot feel them. Alternatively, if they are opting for a natural birth, they will want these muscles to work quickly and effectively when it comes time to push.

Learning how to do ujjayi breathing primes the mom-to-be for labour and childbirth by training them to stay calm when they need it most. When a person is in pain or afraid, their body produces adrenalin and may decrease the production of oxytocin, a hormone that makes labour progress. A regular yoga practice will help the mom-to-be to fight the urge to tighten up when they feel pain, and show them how to relax instead.

Me time

Some women say that attending yoga is the only time in the week that they truly have for themselves during the pregnancy, especially when they have a toddler at home.

Meet new friends

It is not uncommon for a woman to feel isolated during pregnancy. By attending a prenatal yoga class, you can meet other women who are going through the same changes mentally, physically, and emotionally. You can draw from the wealth of experience in the class. This is especially important for first-time mamas.

Yoga poses to avoid and modify

Even if you are going to prenatal yoga classes, it is critical that you let your instructor know that you are pregnant, what trimester you are in, and if you are new to yoga. Many postures are not appropriate for pregnant women and there are modifications which make the recommended postures more comfortable and safe.

In general, you should always listen to your body and stop doing any pose that feels uncomfortable, even it if it a pose that is safe for pregnant women. Acknowledge any feelings of pain or discomfort and make the required adjustments or modifications to the posture as needed, there is no reason to push through a pose that is making you feel uncomfortable.

Inversions

If you are pregnant you should avoid inverted postures such as headstands and shoulder stands. You are at risk of tearing or straining muscles because of the pregnancy hormones (relaxin) flowing through your veins. Relaxin allows the uterus to expand but it also causes connective tissue to soften. You do not want to encourage blood to flow away from the uterus. If it feels OK, you can try legs up the wall.

Move slowly

Your yoga movements should be slow and meditative to avoid light-headedness. Your center of gravity is changing a little every day so your balance may not be as solid as you are used to. You do not want to tip head below the heart in 3rd trimester.

Do not over stretch

Be aware of "Gumby syndrome." The extra dose of relaxin in your body may give you a false sense of flexibility, leaving you vulnerable to injury. Be mindful of this and be careful not to exceed your normal range of motion.

Stay away from hot classes

It is generally not safe to practice hot yoga or Bikram yoga as it could cause overheating. Stick to classes where the room temperature is 30 degrees Celsius or less.

Make space for baby

Squishing your baby feels really restrictive and uncomfortable. When bending forward, hinge from the hips, leading with the breastbone and extending the spine from the crown of the head down to the tailbone. This allows more space for the ribs to move, which makes breathing easier and puts less pressure on the fetus. If the belly is too big for this movement, a yoga strap can be placed behind the feet and held by both hands or ease can be found by placing a rolled-up towel under the buttocks to elevate the body, and open the legs about hip-width apart, to give the belly more room to come forward.

You also want to gently contract the uddiyana bandha, about 10 % rather than the normal 25%.

Avoid deep twists as they compress the internal organs, including the uterus. Try twisting more gently from the shoulders and back than from the waist, to avoid putting any pressure on the abdomen. Or do an open twist, which

means twisting away from the forward leg and smile at your
neighbour.

First Trimester

Many prenatal adaptations are designed to accommodate a
big belly and prevent compression of the uterus. During the
first trimester, the uterus remains fairly small and is protected
by the pelvis, so this is less of an issue. There are not many
restrictions this early in the pregnancy.

Remember to drink lots of fluids before, during and after the
practice to keep your body hydrated. Avoid jarring activities
such as jumping; rather, step feet apart to hip-width or step
feet forward or back in a vinyasa.

Also, it is valuable to breathe deeply and regularly as you
stretch. Avoid any pranayama requiring breath retention or
rapid inhales and exhales. Instead practice the birthing breath;
deep inhales through the nose and exhales through the
mouth.

Second Trimester

During the second trimester it is not recommended that
pregnant women do postures which require them to lie flat on
their backs. The weight of the baby on the uterus compresses
a major vein and can affect the amount of oxygen traveling
back to your heart and to your baby. This can cause dizziness,
shortness of breath and nausea. Savasana can be done lying
on the side with knees bent using bolsters and blankets for
support or you can do a seated meditation. Once you are
starting to show, postures which require lying on the belly
should be avoided.

Your joints are beginning to loosen up now and your sense of balance is changing, so you need to proceed with caution. It is recommended that you don't try to hold poses for a long time.

You may want to ease up on poses like boat pose or plank that use the abdominal muscles because they have a lot of stretching to do to accommodate your growing belly. Ideally your abs will soften. You can get your abs back on track after baby is born.

Third Trimester

With the belly growing bigger each day in the third trimester, pregnant women are probably feeling less graceful. It is wise to perform standing poses with your heels to the wall or using a chair or the wall for support to avoid losing your balance and risking injury. Props such as blocks and straps can also help you move through different poses with greater stability.

It is especially important now to not hold poses for a long time; but rather to keep moving. If you feel any discomfort, you should stop.

Avoid deep backbends as they stretch the entire front of the torso. If done near the end of the pregnancy the belly can stretch excessively making it more difficult to return to normal shape after delivery.

Guest Authors

Margot Schelew

Margot Schelew works towards helping people find ease and happiness in their life. She motivates and inspires all those who come in contact with her. She has been doing this for many years as a yoga instructor, and now takes it to a higher level with Hypnosis in the City, her hypnotherapy business. She is also delighted to be teaching HypnoBirthing - The Mongan Method prenatal classes.

When Margot was in the middle of her child bearing years (in the 80's) she went to Kripalu Institute for a number of yoga workshops. She brought the knowledge home with her and practiced regularly after her children were in bed. She remembers falling asleep in the child pose and in the reclined hero pose a number of times. As she left her house to go to her yoga class, her girls (that's me!) would hang off her legs like boat anchors... but she went just the same. She luxuriated in the stretches and then promptly fell asleep in Savasana every time.

Being pregnant was a very positive experience for Margot. In fact, at times she would be walking down the street with her baby (me!) in her arms and see a pregnant woman walk by, and feel envious... knowing that she had the delivery to look forward to and holding a brand new baby! Is there any experience in a woman's life that could rank higher on the scale of euphoria?

As a yoga teacher and HypnoBirthing instructor she looks forward to guiding pregnant women through the yoga breathing techniques and relaxation exercises with compassion and inspiration.

Check out her website hypnosisinthecity.ca

Andrea Ashley

Andrea Ashley is all about Clinical Aromatherapy, Custom Skin Care, and inspiring more self-love and kindness in the world.

Andrea Ashley has an education in advanced skincare, master clinical aromatherapy, diplomas in both organic skincare science and organic skincare formulation and certifications in holistic therapies. She has brought her passions together to create a brand that is kind to our skin and bodies, but most of, all that INSPIRE people to be kind to themselves and to each other.

Andrea Ashley's products are all focused on aromatherapy and custom skin care. What this means is that her site is for the DIYers, the formulators or the people who want a custom product created specific to their needs. This is to encourage people to really take their self-care and skin care into their own hands. We are all different and our beauty and health needs are as well, so customization is of utmost importance to her.

Andrea Ashley Essential oils and raw ingredients are available for retail, wholesale and bulk, and for private label should you wish to have your own branded line.

Contact her at hello@andreaashley.ca to discuss how she can design a signature product or recommend essential oils just for you and your holistic needs.

Check out her website andreaashley.ca

<u>Want More?</u>

I love to play in the kitchen and have created countless holistically delicious recipes that accommodate a wide variety of food allergies, diets and lifestyle choices.

My healthy recipes are made with whole food ingredients that promote health and wellness. Most of my cookbooks are available in digital format and print.

<u>Healthy Fresh Salads</u>

Have you ever found yourself thinking "I need to be more creative with veggies"?

This is a common complaint I hear a lot from my clients and readers.

Everyone knows they need to be eating lots of veggies, but the thought of eating another salad made with lettuce from a bag and store bought dressing makes everyone want to yawn with boredom.

That is why I created Jesse Lane Wellness Cookbook: Healthy Fresh Salads. It contains over 30 exciting and fresh gluten-free salad recipes. The recipes are all "fresh", not only are they created using fresh veggies, but they are also inspired, creative and anything but boring.

https://www.jesselanewellness.com/healthy-fresh-salads/

<u>Healthy Homemade Soups & Sandwiches</u>

Are you looking for a nutrient-dense meal that is super cheap?

Soup is a super inexpensive way to get more veggies and nutrients into your diet. It is packed with healing herbs that can reduce inflammation, ease digestion, and provide antioxidant support. Studies have found that soup consumption can even help with weight management!

Jesse Lane Wellness Cookbook: Healthy Homemade Soups & Sandwiches contains over 30 holistically delicious soup and sandwich recipes (with stunning images) that are easy to prepare.

It also contains information of how to properly freeze and reheat soups, explains the downfalls of canned soups, and provides the nutritional breakdown of fresh, frozen and canned veggies.

https://www.jesselanewellness.com/healthy-homemade-soups-sandwiches/

<u>Healthy Dairy Free Desserts</u>

Do you want to have your cake and eat it too? Now you can!

Jesse Lane Wellness Cookbook: Healthy Dairy Free Desserts contains over 30 holistically delicious dessert recipes (with stunning images) that you can enjoy guilt-free!

All of the unique recipes are nutritionist approved, made with whole food ingredients and do not contain any soy, dairy, white flour or processed sugar.

Healthy Dairy Free Desserts also contains a guide to healthy baking substitutes and alternative sugars, so you can learn how to turn your family favourites into healthy desserts.

https://www.jesselanewellness.com/dairy-free-desserts/

<u>21 Day smoothie Guide</u>

Want to jump on the smoothie bandwagon but don't know where to start?

Recently, smoothies have been all the rage with everyone and their grandma making them in effort to improve their health. The problem is you might be making common smoothie mistakes and creating a drink that is not only unhealthy but contributing to weight gain!

Holistic in the City 21 Day Smoothie Guide contains 21 delicious smoothie recipes made with love by 7 Holistic Nutritionists. It also has lots of information including our basic smoothie formula, the answer to the age-old debate of juicing vs smoothies and what to look for when buying protein powder.

https://www.jesselanewellness.com/holistic-city-21-day-smoothie-guide/

Let's Get Social

You can connect with me on Facebook, Instagram, and Twitter as @jesselwellness and I'm also on YouTube.

I always get so excited when someone makes one of my recipes or tries my healthy living advice and tags me in the picture!!!

Website: http://www.jesselanewellness.com/

Facebook: http://www.facebook.com/JesseLWellness

Instagram: http://instagram.com/jesselwellness

Twitter: https://twitter.com/JesseLWellness

YouTube:
http://www.youtube.com/c/JesseLaneWellnesscom

References

1. Haas, Elson M., and Buck Levin. Staying Healthy with Nutrition: The Complete Guide to Diet and Nutritional Medicine. Berkeley: Celestial Arts, 2006. Print. http://amzn.to/2undcXA

2. Balch, Phyllis A. Prescription for Nutritional Healing. New York: Avery, a Member of Penguin Group (USA), 2010. Print. http://amzn.to/2tQwtNX

3. Mateljan, George. The World's Healthiest Foods: Essential Guide for the Healthiest Way of Eating. Seattle, WA: George Mateljan Foundation, 2007. Print. http://amzn.to/2vh2q1e

4. Hoffman, David. Holistic Herbal: A Safe and Practical Guide to Making and Using Herbal Remedies. London: Thorsons, 2002. Print. http://amzn.to/2tQn20F

5. Skillins, Susan. Nutrition Through The Lifespan. Institute of Holistic Nutrition, Toronto. 2012. Nutrition for Pregnancy and Lactation Lecture.

6. Naturally Designed Pregnancy & Early Childhood. Institute of Holistic Nutrition, Toronto. 2012. Slides and Course Notes.

7. Loy, S. L., M. Marhazlina, Y. N. Azwany, and J. M. Hamid. "Higher Intake of Fruits and Vegetables in Pregnancy Is Associated with Birth Size." The Southeast Asian Journal of Tropical Medicine and Public Health. U.S. National Library of Medicine, Sept. 2011. Web. 13 July 2017.

8. Ramón, R., F. Ballester, C. Iñiguez, M. Rebagliato, M. Murcia, A. Esplugues, A. Marco, M. García, and J. Vioque. "Vegetable but Not Fruit Intake during Pregnancy Is Associated with Newborn Anthropometric Measures." The Journal of Nutrition. U.S. National Library of Medicine, Mar. 2009. Web. 13 July 2017.

9. Shukla, S., R. Mathur, and A. O. Prakash. "Antifertility Profile of the Aqueous Extract of Moringa Oleifera Roots." Journal of Ethnopharmacology. U.S. National Library of Medicine, Jan. 1988. Web. 13 July 2017.

10. Araújo, L. C., J. S. Aguiar, T. H. Napoleão, F. V. Mota, A. L. Barros, M. C. Moura, M. C. Coriolano, L. C. Coelho, T. G. Silva, and P. M. Paiva. "Evaluation of Cytotoxic and Anti-inflammatory Activities of Extracts and Lectins from Moringa Oleifera Seeds." PloS One. U.S. National Library of Medicine, 09 Dec. 2013. Web. 13 July 2017.

11. Bose, Chinmoy K. "Possible Role of Moringa Oleifera Lam. Root in Epithelial Ovarian Cancer." Medscape General Medicine. Medscape, 2007. Web. 13 July 2017.

12. Nakano, S., H. Takekoshi, and M. Nakano. "Chlorella (Chlorella Pyrenoidosa) Supplementation Decreases Dioxin and Increases Immunoglobulin a Concentrations in Breast Milk." Journal of Medicinal Food. U.S. National Library of Medicine, Mar. 2007. Web. 13 July 2017.

13. Teran, E., I. Hernandez, B. Nieto, R. Tavara, J. E. Ocampo, and A. Calle. "Coenzyme Q10 Supplementation during Pregnancy Reduces the Risk of Pre-eclampsia." International Journal of Gynaecology and Obstetrics: The Official Organ of the International Federation of Gynaecology and Obstetrics. U.S. National Library of Medicine, Apr. 2009. Web. 13 July 2017.

14. Gallo Gideon Koren, Michael, MD. "Can Herbal

Products Be Used Safely during Pregnancy?:Focus on Echinacea." Motherisk. The Hospital for Sick Children (SickKids), Sept. 2001. Web. 13 July 2017.

15. Benson, Jonathan. "Radiation doctor says TSA naked body scanners can cause cancer." NaturalNews. N.p., 5 Jan. 2012. Web. 21 July 2017.

16. Tisserand, Robert, and Rodney Young. Essential oil safety: a guide for health care professionals. Edinburgh: Churchill Livingstone/Elsevier, 2014. Print.

17. Schnaubelt, Kurt. Medical aromatherapy: healing with essential oils. Berkeley, CA: Frog, 1999. Print. http://amzn.to/2u5LaLp

18. Parker, Susan. Power of the Seed: Your Guide to Oils for Health & Beauty. Port Townsend: WA: Process Media, 2014. Print. http://amzn.to/2vQZQ2W

19. Romm, Aviva Jill. The natural pregnancy book: your complete guide to a safe, organic pregnancy and childbirth with herbs, nutrition, and other holistic choices. Berkeley: Ten Speed Press, 2014. Print. http://amzn.to/2wg3B1m

Index